Hot Topics in Acute Care Surgery and Trauma

This series covers the most debated issues in acute care and trauma surgery, from perioperative management to organizational and health policy issues. Since 2011, the founder members of the World Society of Emergency Surgery's (WSES) Acute Care and Trauma Surgeons group, who endorse the series, realized the need to provide more educational tools for young surgeons in training and for general physicians and other specialists new to this discipline: WSES is currently developing a systematic scientific and educational program founded on evidence-based medicine and objective experience. Covering the complex management of acute trauma and non-trauma surgical patients, this series makes a significant contribution to this program and is a valuable resource for both trainees and practitioners in acute care surgery.

Marco Ceresoli • Fikri M. Abu-Zidan
Kristan L. Staudenmayer • Fausto Catena
Federico Coccolini
Editors

Statistics and Research Methods for Acute Care and General Surgeons

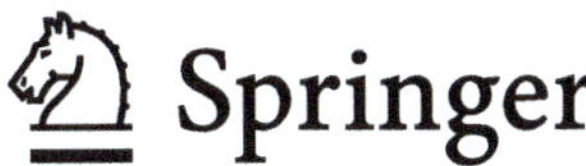

Editors
Marco Ceresoli
General and Emergency Surgery
Department, School of Medicine and
Surgery, Milano-Bicocca University
Monza, Italy

Kristan L. Staudenmayer
Department of Surgery, Stanford University
Stanford, CA, USA

Federico Coccolini
Department of General, Emergency and
Trauma Surgery, Pisa University Hospital
Pisa, Pisa, Italy

Fikri M. Abu-Zidan
Department of Surgery, College of
Medicine and Health Science
United Arab Emirates University
Abu Dhabi, United Arab Emirates

Fausto Catena
General and Emergency Surgery
Department Bufalini Hospital
Cesena, Italy

ISSN 2520-8284 ISSN 2520-8292 (electronic)
Hot Topics in Acute Care Surgery and Trauma
ISBN 978-3-031-13820-1 ISBN 978-3-031-13818-8 (eBook)
https://doi.org/10.1007/978-3-031-13818-8

This Springer imprint is published by the registered company Springer Nature Switzerland AG
The registered company address is: Gewerbestrasse 11, 6330 Cham, Switzerland

Preface: Why a Statistics Manual in the Series of "Hot Topics in Acute Care Surgery"?

In the last decades we have experienced major medical and surgical advancements. The transition from "*eminence-based medicine*" to "*evidence-based medicine*" is one of the most important pillars of modern medicine. Fortunately, it is now extremely rare to hear odious terms reflecting personal opinions like "*we have always done it that way*" or "*my mentor taught me that…*". and it is now recognized that clinical decisions should be made according to the evidence.

The ability to read and properly understand scientific research articles is vital to employ an evidence-based medicine approach. How many times we have blindly trusted the results of a paper without critically evaluating it? We find ourselves surprised later on to find that these results were flawed or wrongly interpreted. The modern healthcare professionals, including acute care surgeons, must have the essential skills to practice evidence-based medicine which includes the ability to design a research project and perform statistical analyses.

In the famous Italian novel *the Adventures of Pinocchio* by C. Collodi, the wooden marionette Pinocchio meets two shady characters, the fox and the cat, who try to cheat him by taking advantage of his trust. We think that this is similar to a young surgeon who reads a paper trusting its reported p-values without understanding, interpreting, and critically appraising what was reported.

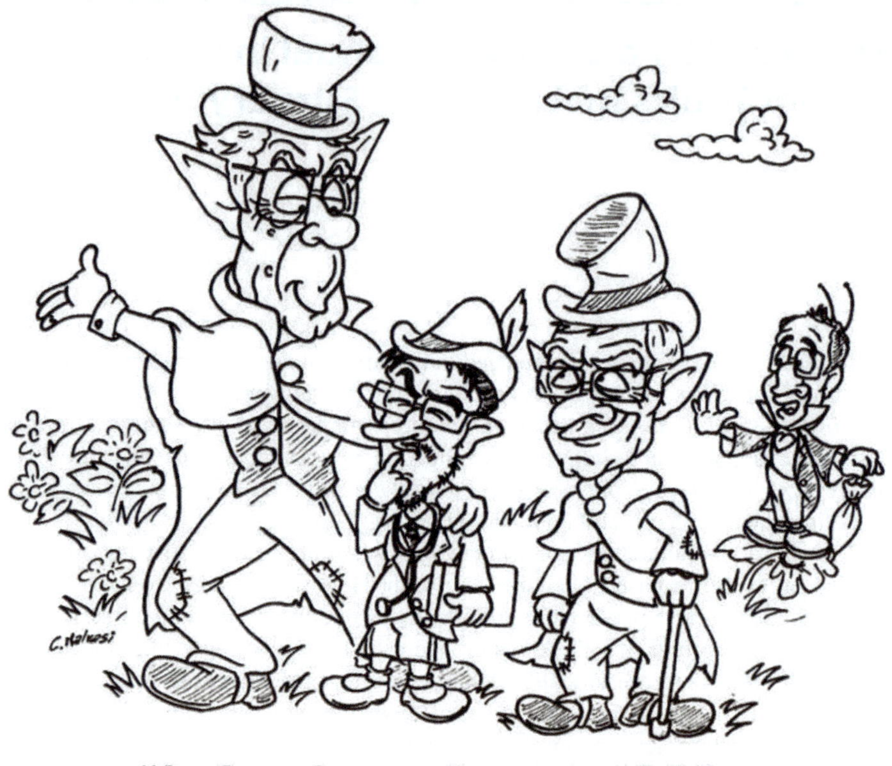

"look at the p-value: it's <0.05

We therefore have decided to write this concise manual with the goal of helping to strengthen the acute care surgeon's statistical knowledge and to provide the necessary support to face the complexity of evidence-based medicine.

Some acute care surgeons may attempt to use a classical statistical book to interpret and analyze the data from their studies. They might get discouraged when they encounter statistical concepts expressed as complex mathematical formulas. This makes the surgeon entirely dependent on a statistician who may not have the same clinical understanding or the context for the clinical problem.

We have designed this manual to be an easy-to-use reference for acute care surgeons. It has been written by surgeons for surgeons with straightforward explanations and examples, without math. It is meant to improve a surgeon's basic understanding of applied statistics, rather than a deep dive into theoretical statistics. By doing so, we hope to make statistics more accessible and expect that readers will find that fundamental statistical principles can be easy to understand.

The present manual has three parts. The first covers scientific methods as applied to medical research. The second covers basic statistics. The third covers commonly used advanced statistical methods such as multivariate analysis, meta-analysis, and survival analysis. These chapters will provide practical examples in order to provide context and to ease readers into statistical science.

Monza, Italy	Marco Ceresoli
Abu Dhabi, United Arab Emirates	Fikri M. Abu-Zidan
Stanford, CA, USA	Kristan L. Staudenmayer
Cesena, Italy	Fausto Catena
Pisa, Italy	Federico Coccolini

Contents

Part I

Designing Your Research

Study Typology: An Overview

1

Giacomo Mulinacci and Marco Carbone

1.1 Introduction

Choosing the right study type is the first, fundamental, and often limiting step in the publication of a scientific paper. Before submitting a paper to a scientific journal, several factors should be cautiously considered to limit the risk of study failure. This chapter represents an overview of different research studies, with a particular focus on the indications, major pro and cons of each study type.

G. Mulinacci · M. Carbone (✉)
Division of Gastroenterology, Department of Medicine and Surgery, University of Milano-Bicocca, Milan, Italy

Center for Autoimmune Liver Diseases, European Reference Network (ERN) RARE-LIVER Center, San Gerardo Hospital, ASST Monza, Monza, Italy
e-mail: g.mulinacci@campus.unimib.it; marco.carbone@unimib.it

M. Ceresoli et al. (eds.), *Statistics and Research Methods for Acute Care and General Surgeons*, Hot Topics in Acute Care Surgery and Trauma,
https://doi.org/10.1007/978-3-031-13818-8_1

1.2 The Need for Evidence-Based Medicine

Progression of human knowledge is obtained through the continuous generation and accumulation of measurable and testable data. This is the basis of scientific research. Medical research is a branch of scientific research that embraces various fields, including medicine, biology, chemistry, and pharmacology. It aims to improve the knowledge about human species and its environment, with the goal to fight diseases by developing or repurposing drugs or medical procedures. Research studies should be conducted to guarantee the dignity and the well-being of study participants while ensuring minimal risks.

The concept of evidence-based medicine (EBM), largely debated in the last decades, is now widely recognized as having a fundamental role in research. Its definition dates to 1991, when Gordon Guyatt, a Canadian physician and academic, coined the term in a short editorial for the ACP Journal Club [1]. EBM was defined as "the conscientious, explicit, and judicious use of current best evidence in making decisions about the care of individual patients." The practice of EBM is a continuous combination of scientific research and clinician personal expertise, acquired through daily clinical practice.

1.3 Research Studies

Decades of research in the scientific field led to the development of a broad spectrum of study typologies, and the choice of the appropriate experimental design represents a critical step. Study quality, accuracy, and likelihood of being published are all strongly influenced by the selection of a proper study design. Even if each study type contributes to the growth of scientific knowledge, some have a higher impact than others (Fig. 1.1).

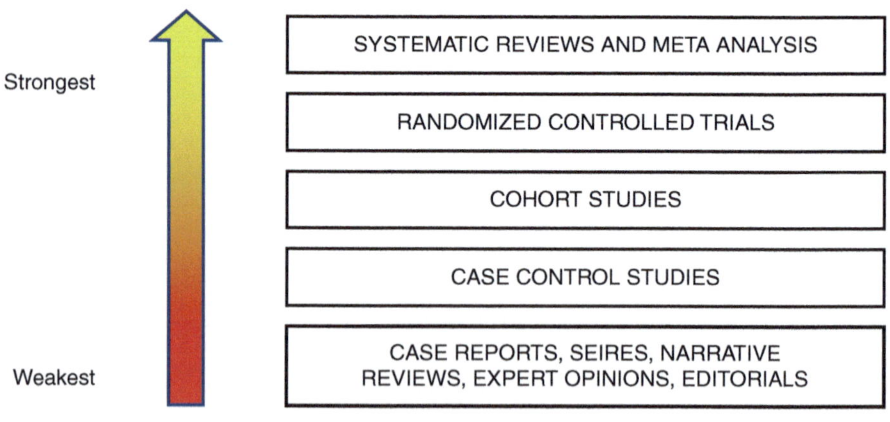

Fig. 1.1 Hierarchy of level of evidence of different study types

The main distinction of study designs is between *primary* vs. *secondary* study types, even if they can be also divided into *descriptive* vs. *analytical* and *observational* vs. *experimental.*

When approaching different research studies, the first macroscopic distinction is between primary and secondary study types. The major difference between them is the active participation of authors in data collection, which is a prerequisite of primary studies. Secondary research, also known as desk research, gathers information and data from already conducted and published studies.

Within descriptive studies, researchers observe and describe the data, without performing any statistical analysis. They report the distribution of diseases or health-related concerns in different populations, without seeking the link between exposure and outcome. They are observational in nature, and they primarily evaluate features like disease prevalence and incidence. Even if they occupy one of the lowest rungs in the hierarchy of clinical studies, they can be relevant for the possibility to illustrate novel, unusual features identified during medical practice [2]. Despite this, the absence of corroborative data questioned their utility, since they often rise scientific questions that are not sustained on further research [3].

Analytical studies seek and try to quantify correlations between exposure and outcome. Differently from descriptive studies, they can be both observational or experimental, depending on whether the exposure is determined by the nature or assigned by an investigator. Observational studies are a pure description and collection of information about populations, diseases, beliefs, or behaviors. Experimental studies require human intervention.

1.4 Primary and Secondary Research Studies

1.4.1 Primary Studies

Primary research studies can be laboratorial, clinical, and epidemiological, even if the distinction is not always well delineated. This chapter mainly focuses on the clinical and epidemiological studies that represent the "daily bread" for clinicians.

1.4.1.1 Laboratorial Research

Laboratorial research, also called basic or experimental, has the aim to acquire novel knowledge or principles to better understand natural phenomena. It raises new questions and ways of thinking with a revolutionary potential, and it fulfills the sense of curiosity, intrinsic of all scientists, through the development of new ideas, concepts, and hypothesis, which set the basis for scientific progress. Basic research is often carried out on cellular or animal samples, and it represents the starting point for clinical and epidemiological research. It can be used as a preliminarily assessment of the physio-pathologic mechanisms and/or therapeutic effects of a novel agent.

It hardly helps clinicians with daily concerns, since rigorous and long-lasting controls are necessary for their knowledge to be concretely accessible. This might take up to a few decades [4].

1.4.1.2 Clinical Studies

Clinical studies consist of the collection of information from patients, diseases, or responses to different treatments with the aim of developing novel therapies, methods, prognostic scores. Differently from basic research, the human being is the target of clinical research. Clinical studies are further divided into observational (non-interventional) and experimental (interventional).

Clinical Observational Studies

Clinical observational studies (COS) are descriptive, retrospective studies characterized by the absence of a direct action from the investigators, who passively observe the effect of a risk factor, diagnostic test, or treatment without intervening. They can be conducted on small or large populations, and they enable to examine the natural course of different diseases. A major advantage of COS is that study participants, being retrospectively followed, never alter their behavior. This feature enables COS to assess the natural course of several disorders, thus supporting clinicians with real-life clinical data, possibly indicating to clinicians how major experimental trials can translate to clinical practice [5].

Case Reports and Case Series

Case reports and series are the simplest and most common among COS since they describe clinical phenomena occurring in up to few patients. They usually describe an atypical manifestation of a particular disease, an unexpected treatment response, unique medical or surgical approaches, or novel findings of a disease which might provide a hint on its pathogenesis. Case series are an aggregation of several similar cases. Some authors accept three cases to be a case series, therefore the boundary between case reports and series is subtle [6].

COS, in particular case series, can help to collect initial information from rare diseases, for which is hard to collect large numbers. As case reports and series predominantly describe rare events or findings, their citation index is inferior to other study typologies(Table 1.1). This largely restricts their likelihood to be accepted and published in highly impacting international journals.

Table 1.1 Main features of different study typologies

Study type	Prospective vs. retrospective	Difficulty	Costs	Sample size	LOE	Major strengths	Major weaknesses
Case report	Retrospective	+	Low	1–3 patients	+	• Easy and fast • Offers novel observations and generate hypothesis • Flexible structure	• Causal inference and generalization not possible • Risk for result overinterpretation • Selection bias towards positive results
Case series	Retrospective	+	Low	Few patients	+	Same as case reports	Same as case reports
Narrative reviews	Retrospective	++	Low	Largely variable, no upper or lower limits	+	• Easy and fast • Increases the overall knowledge about a topic • Identifies gaps in the existing literature	• Selection bias towards positive results • Lack of systematic assessment
Cross-sectional	Retrospective	++	Low-medium	Few hundred-few thousand	++	• Relatively easy and quick • Identifies disease prevalence • Assessment of multiple outcomes and exposures	• Temporal association between exposure and outcome difficult to be determined • Inability to assess incidence • Not suitable for rare disorders
Case–control	Retrospective	++	Low-medium	Few hundreds	+++	• Relatively easy and fast • Assessment of rare disorders	• Selection bias • Unable to determine disease incidence

(continued)

Table 1.1 (continued)

Study type	Prospective vs. retrospective	Difficulty	Costs	Sample size	LOE	Major strengths	Major weaknesses
Cohort	Retrospective or prospective	++	Medium-high	Few hundred-few thousand	+++	• Relatively easy and fast • Assess multiple outcomes for a given exposure • Assessment of rare disorders	• Selection bias • Large numbers required for rare exposures
Ecological	Retrospective	++	Medium	Few hundred-few thousand	+++	• Relatively easy and fast • Assessment of exposure data at area rather than individual levels • Assessment of spatial framework of disease and exposure	• Lack of individual data assessment
Clinical trials	Prospective	+++	High	Varies between single phases	++++	• Minimize the confounders • Avoid selection bias	• Ethical issues • Time consuming • Risk for study dropout
Systematic reviews +/− meta-analysis	Retrospective	+++	Low	No limits of study considered	++++	• Resume the best available research evidence about a topic • Transparency of each phase of the construction	• Selection bias • Author interpretation of summarized results

LOE level of evidence

Clinical Experimental Studies

Clinical experimental studies include clinical trials and epidemiological studies. Clinical trials are prospective studies primarily aimed at evaluating the efficacy (a measure of the success in an artificial setting), effectiveness (a measure of the value in the real world), and safety of a medical and/or behavioral intervention on large-scale groups. They are among the studies with the highest level of evidence available in research and the most effective study typology to assess the efficacy of a novel intervention or treatment, thus enhancing the value of health care provided. They require the approval from local ethical committees, after a thorough assessment of the risk-to-benefit ratio of the specific study. They focus on highly specific research questions supported by previous evidence. Among clinical trials, a further distinction occurs between single-arm, placebo-controlled, crossover, factorial, and noninferiority trials [7].

Each patient enrolled in a clinical trial must sign an informed consent that should clearly and extensively explain the purpose, duration, risks, and benefits of the intervention. Further, it should be specified that participation in the study is voluntary, and that dropout can occur at any time point and would not change the patient's care [8].

A pivotal step in the design of a clinical trial is the selection of study participants, both healthy and diseased, that should be representative of the general population. Unfortunately, this is often limited by several requirements, scientific and non-scientific, that might introduce potential selection confounders [9].

Study participants should meet a certain sample size, to successfully address study questions with sufficient statistical power, defined as the likelihood of at least 80% to correctly identify statistically significant differences between outcomes of interventions, when it is clinically detectable [10, 11].

Another important momentum in the construction of clinical trials is the choice of endpoints that should represent outcomes or events that enable an objective assessment of the effect of a medical intervention (drug or other agents). Clinical endpoints are generally classified as primary, secondary, or tertiary. Primary endpoints specifically address the research question, towards which the trial is designed. They strictly depend upon the population of interest, disease characteristics, and treatment aim. They can be single or multiple and often represent hard clinical outcomes, such as death, survival, or cure. However, some endpoints might be difficult to measure (eg. quality of life), expensive, or might require long time and large sample sizes, particularly for diseases with a slow progression (e.g., chronic liver diseases). In such cases, surrogate endpoints are used, which are a measure of effect of a specific treatment that may correlate with a real clinical endpoint but does not necessarily have a guaranteed relationship. To be considered reliable, putative surrogate endpoints must undergo a meticulous process of validation, with the aim of confirming their association with the primary outcome.

Secondary endpoints are additional events of interest that should be pre-determined in the study protocol, and towards which the study is not powered. They are usually addressed in smaller sub-groups of the entire population, and their analysis should be cautiously interpreted. Due to their lower statistical relevance, they

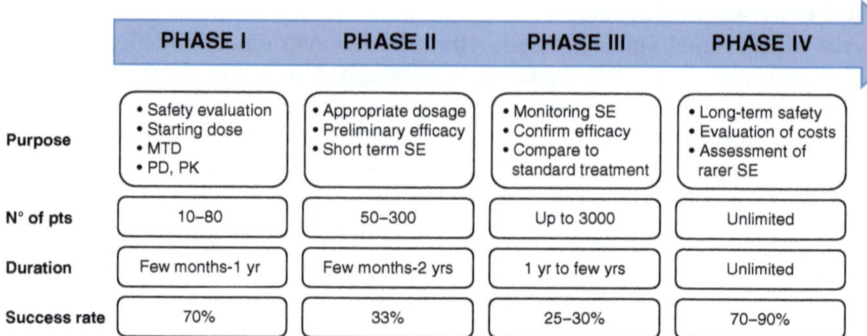

Fig. 1.2 Main features of different phases of randomized controlled trials. *MTD* minimum tolerated dose, *PD* pharmacodynamics, *PK* pharmacokinetics, *SE* side effects

are generally used to support results from primary endpoints or to provide information for future research. Tertiary endpoints are rarely assessed and usually describe rarer outcomes.

Clinical trials are generally divided into 4 phases, designed with the primary aim of ensuring the safety of study participants. The major characteristics of each phase are represented in Fig. 1.2.

Phase I clinical trials estimate, for each novel agent, the safety, starting dose, maximum tolerated dose, dose-escalation method, pharmacological and metabolic properties, and eventual interactions with other drugs. Being the first approach of a new drug or intervention to patients, phase I clinical trials are designed with a limited number of healthy or diseased volunteers and are often conducted as open label studies, with both investigators and participants aware of the treatment administered. The assessment of the maximum tolerated dose of an agent is often difficult since the trial should be designed to limit the exposure of too many patients to subtherapeutic doses of the drug while preserving safety. This can be achieved through different escalation methods.

It is important to limit the patient misperception that the drug tested during phase I might lead to direct health improvement. This is particularly true for trials testing drugs in refractory or end-stage disorders (i.e., chemotherapeutic agents for oncologic patients), and it can be prevented through the distribution of adequate informed consent forms.

Successful phase I trials are followed by phase II trials. They are exploratory trials conducted on few volunteer patients with the disease of interest. The number of patients can vary, even if it is usually higher than phase I. Phase II trials assess the preliminary efficacy and the appropriate dose of the drug, other than further deepening the issues of drug safety, pharmacokinetics, and pharmacodynamics. In other words, they evaluate whether it has sufficient activity to warrant further development and access to phase III. They might also tackle essential questions for phase III trials (i.e., drug dosages, posology, and route of administration).

Phase III clinical trials test a potential treatment on a large scale and represent the best tool to consolidate new treatment approaches. They confirm the efficacy and estimate the incidence of common adverse effects, defined as those occurring at a rate not lower than 1 over 100 people [12]. Among type III clinical trials, the comparative trial is the most common. It compares the targeted drug with a placebo or a conventional treatment. To calculate the sample size of a comparative trial, several design parameters must be considered. Saad et al. summarized them within the ABCDE rule [13], where "A" stands for "α" and it represents the significance level, or type I error rate (the probability that the trial will show a treatment effect when it does not have any), which is usually below 5%; "B" stands for β, and it represents the type II error (the probability that the trial will not show an effect of a treatment that actually has an effect), usually $\leq$20%; "C" and "E" represent the outcome of control and experimental groups, respectively. Both groups rely on disease type, trial endpoint, and patient selection; the outcome in the experimental group also depends on treatment efficacy. Finally, "D" stands for the dropout rate.

Interim analysis, both planned and unplanned, can be performed during phase III trials to evaluate the possibility of early declaration of success or unsuccess of an intervention. They can also suggest modification in sample size or study design. They are often conducted by an Independent Data Monitoring Committee.

Prior to enter phase IV, Food and Drug Administration (FDA) approval must occur. It is often required that several phase III trials are conducted prior to entering phase IV, which represents the terminal step of drug approval, and it is often required by regulatory authorities or by sponsoring companies. The aim of phase IV trials is to identify rarer side effects, long-term safety surveillance, and to evaluate cost of the intervention. Negative side effects during phase IV trials may lead to drug removal from the market or to restricted use.

An exception to this stepwise authorization process occurs when the benefits of a rapid approval outweigh the risks, as it occurs for rare disorders with unmet clinical needs or for emergency situation, with a recent example of the SARS-CoV-2 pandemic. In such cases, the European Medicine Agency (EMA) can release a conditional marketing authorization to speed up drug approval [14]. Conditionally approved agents still require phase IV trials to assess for long-term side effects.

1.4.1.3 Epidemiological Research

Epidemiological research deals with disease patterns, causes, incidence, prevalence, and control within a population. It often involves large populations, with good chances to determine the eventual association between exposure and outcomes. Epidemiological studies include case–control, cross-sectional, cohort, and ecological studies.

Cross-Sectional Studies

Cross-sectional studies are retrospective studies that can fit both into the descriptive and analytical group, depending on whether they provide estimates of prevalence of

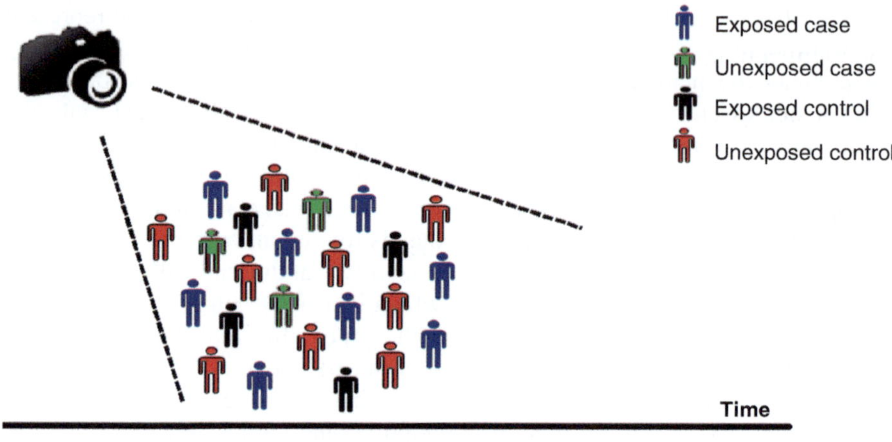

Fig. 1.3 Cross-sectional studies: a snapshot is taken of a particular group of people at a given point in time

disease, or evaluate associations between different parameters. Most commonly, they simultaneously measure exposure and outcome of determined health-related phenomena among the study participants, and patient selection follows previously established inclusion and exclusion criteria. Cross-sectional studies often compare differences of outcomes between exposed and unexposed patients, by taking a one-time snapshot of exposure and outcome (Fig. 1.3). The ability to collect information of a large number of patients in a small amount of time confers them a major role in the evaluation of disease burden of a specific population, thus aiding the description of disease prevalence (either point prevalence or period prevalence), incidence, and geographic or temporal variation of diseases in clinic-based samples. As it occurred for case reports and case series, they can raise scientific hypothesis to be verified with more complex study types. Being a real-life snapshot, cross-sectional studies are prone to several biases, both derived from inappropriate patient selection and physician/laboratory measurement errors. Another limit of these study designs includes the impossibility to determine causal and temporal associations between exposure and outcomes since several intercurrent factors might have influenced this relationship.

Case–Control Studies

Case–control studies are retrospective, observational studies in which two groups with different outcomes are compared based on some supposed causal attribute. They are indeed commonly used to look at factors associated with diseases or outcomes. The selection of study participants in case–control studies is based on the outcome status (Fig. 1.4). Investigators address the past exposure to suspected etiological factors among selected patients and compare it with that of healthy controls. A difficult step in this type of study is the choice of adequate cases and controls. A "case" is a set of criteria used to decide if an individual has a particular disease. Selection of cases should be done to reduce as possible the risk of bias, and choosing the same source (hospitals, clinics, registers, or population) might be of help.

Cohort Studies

Participants of cohort studies are selected and followed up upon the exposure status to something (i.e., a noxious agent, drug, etc.) that the investigator considers as being a potential cause for an outcome. Cohort studies are usually prospective even if they can also be retrospective. At baseline, a population of healthy patients is divided into "exposed" and "unexposed" to a determined risk factor (Fig. 1.4). During the follow-up, each enrolled patient might develop the outcome of interest, irrespective of the exposure status. The investigator will then compare both groups, to search for relationships between exposure and outcome, thus assessing whether that specific risk factor has impact on a determined outcome. Overall, this study methodology is easy, rapid to perform, and costless. Other strengths of cohort studies include the possibility to determine multiple outcomes from single exposures; to assess the temporal relationship between exposure and outcome and to study rare exposures (Fig. 1.5).

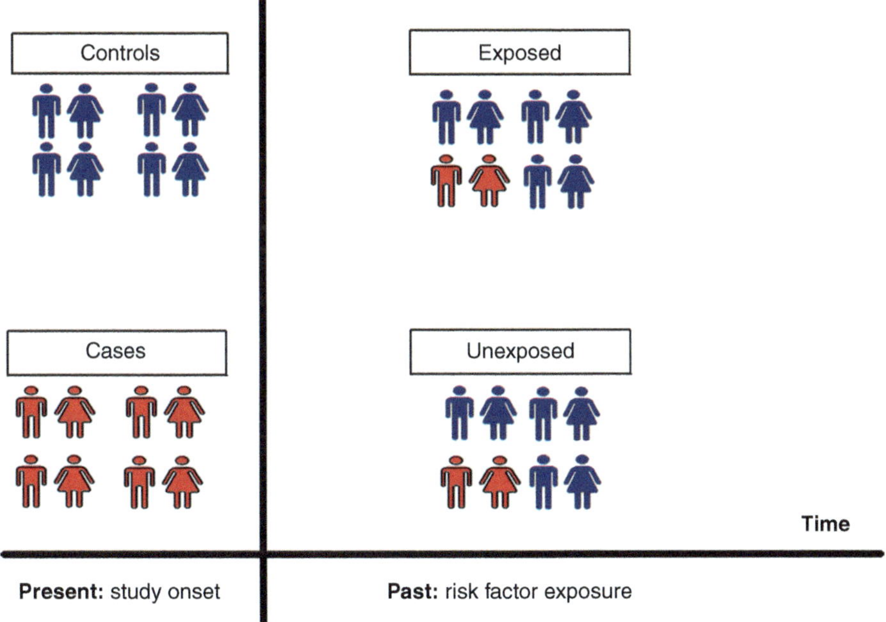

Fig. 1.4 Case–control studies: at day 0 (study onset) patients with a determined condition (cases) are compared with patients without that determined condition (controls) to retrospectively recognize factors that may contribute to the outcome

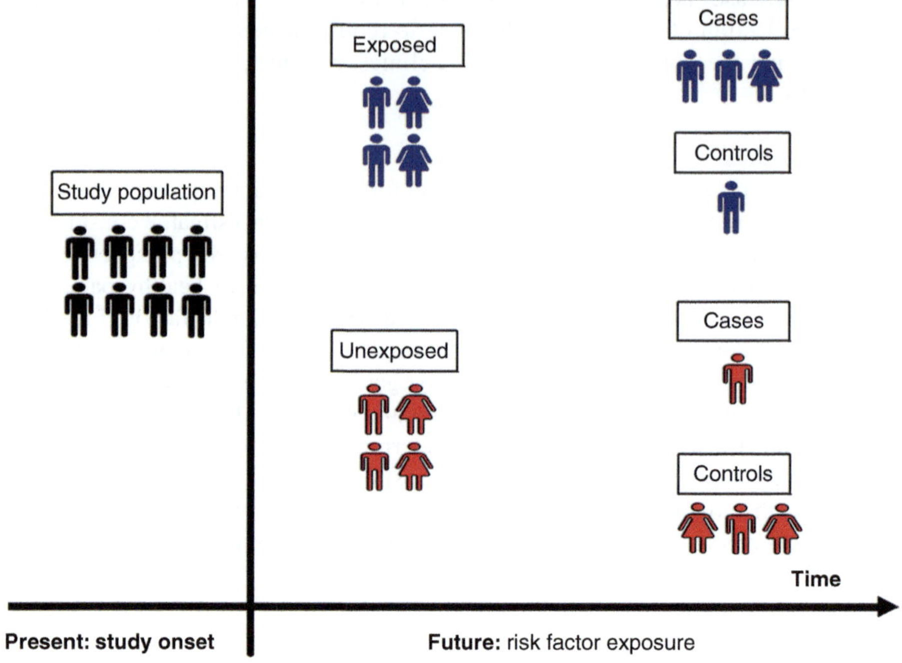

Fig. 1.5 Prospective cohort studies: Healthy patients considered "at risk" upon a specific exposure are followed up in time to identify incident cases

Ecological Studies

An ecologic study focuses to compare groups of people, rather than single individuals. It therefore assesses the overall disease frequency in a population, and it considers the eventual correlation with its average exposure to an agent. The term "ecological" derives from the common use of geographical areas to define the units of analysis. Ecological studies had an important role in the determination of occupational exposure to noxious agents, and they have been used to understand the association of exposure as outcome, as it occurred for selected industrial chemicals with breast cancer incidence in Texas [14].

Other than being cheap and easy to perform, advantages of ecological studies include the possibility to map different pathologies with their risk factors. This is eased by the large number of people possibly included that helps the examination of risk-modifying factors.

1.4.2 Secondary Studies

1.4.2.1 Narrative Reviews

Narrative reviews are among the most frequent type of scientific works in the medical literature. They summarize, describe, and critically analyze the available literature about a topic of interest. As such, they often help clinicians in seeking information about patients care by assembling a great amount of information into a few pages.

Narrative reviews are unstructured, have no pre-set research questions, analysis approach, or protocols. They might be conducted using search words within scientific databases, but without specifying the methods used for selecting and reviewing the literature retrieved [15].

Due to the absence of a-priori protocols and standardized methodologies, authors of narrative reviews freely decide which research works to include. This creates a study selection bias and exposes narrative reviews to large criticisms from experts. Several attempts were made to facilitate the authors to build more valid reviews [16], and a brief scale for quality assessment of narrative review articles has been recently developed, with potential benefits.

1.4.2.2 Systematic Reviews and Meta-Analysis

The worldwide diffusion of Internet led to a rapid surge of scientific information that are made available to everyone. This led to a steep increase in the overall knowledge, but it also made difficult the distinction of high from low quality information.

Systematic reviews assemble the knowledge on a specific topic derived from other study types conducted until that moment, evaluate their reliability and quality, and synthesize their results. The PICO (patient, intervention, comparison, outcome) system is a technic used to start with a clear question to be answered or hypothesis to be tested; perform a comprehensive description of inclusion criteria to limit the bias related to study selection; and attempt to consider the most relevant published and unpublished studies.

They are generally written by experts after a meticulous review of the information gained from both published and unpublished studies.

Meta-analyses are subsets of systematic reviews and can be performed to evaluate the pooled data from two or more different studies to obtain more precise average results. However, if it is not possible to form a pooled estimate, a meta-analysis cannot be performed. As such, all meta-analyses are included in systematic reviews, but the opposite does not always occur.

Both study designs, if well conducted, can be of help to overcome the difficulties associated with the construction of large-scale clinical trials. Appropriate study selection is therefore fundamental, and the Preferred Reporting Items for Systematic Reviews and Meta-Analyses (PRISMA) statement became an important tool for standardization and improvement of the quality of both systematic reviews and meta-analyses [17, 18].

Notwithstanding the use of PRISMA, a major issue of meta-analysis and systematic reports is still linked to publication bias, as often positive and optimistic results are published earlier and on higher impacted journals as compared to unexpected or unpopular ones. This results in the increase of type I errors (high false positive results) in meta-analysis, thus lowering their validity. Efforts are made to limit these biases [19].

Overall, systematic reviews and meta-analysis, together with clinical trials, rank at the top in the hierarchy of evidence (Fig. 1.1) and represent the basis of decision-making in evidence-based medicine.

Third-Party Content No third-party content or material was included in this chapter.

References

1. Guyatt GH. Evidence-based medicine. ACP J Club. 1991:A-16.
2. Aggarwal R, Ranganathan P. Study designs: part 2—descriptive studies. Perspect Clin Res. 2019;10(1):34–6.
3. Hoffman JR. Rethinking case reports. West J Med. 1999;170(5):253–4.
4. Shimomura O. Discovery of green fluorescent protein (GFP) (Nobel lecture). Angew Chem Int Ed Engl. 2009;48(31):5590–602.
5. Ligthelm RJ, Borzì V, Gumprecht J, Kawamori R, Wenying Y, Valensi P. Importance of observational studies in clinical practice. Clin Ther. 2007;29(6 Pt 1):1284–92.
6. Hennekens CH, Buring JE, Mayrent SL. Epidemiology in medicine. Boston, MA: Little, Brown; 1987.
7. Evans SR. Clinical trial structures. J Exp Stroke Transl Med. 2010;3(1):8–18.
8. Gupta UC. Informed consent in clinical research: revisiting few concepts and areas. Perspect Clin Res. 2013;4(1):26–32.
9. Weng C. Optimizing clinical research participant selection with informatics. Trends Pharmacol Sci. 2015;36(11):706–9.
10. Lieber RL. Statistical significance and statistical power in hypothesis testing. J Orthop Res. 1990;8(2):304–9.
11. Umscheid CA, Margolis DJ, Grossman CE. Key concepts of clinical trials: a narrative review. Postgrad Med. 2011;123(5):194–204.
12. Eypasch E, Lefering R, Kum CK, Troidl H. Probability of adverse events that have not yet occurred: a statistical reminder. BMJ. 1995;311(7005):619–20.
13. Saad ED. The ABCDE of sample size calculation. Personal Communication. 2014.
14. Coyle YM, Hynan LS, Euhus DM, Minhajuddin ATM. An ecological study of the association of environmental chemicals on breast cancer incidence in Texas. Breast Cancer Res Treat. 2005;92(2):107–14.
15. Baethge C, Goldbeck-Wood S, Mertens S. SANRA—a scale for the quality assessment of narrative review articles. Res Integr Peer Rev. 2019;4(1):5.
16. Green BN, Johnson CD, Adams A. Writing narrative literature reviews for peer-reviewed journals: secrets of the trade. J Chiropr Med. 2006;5(3):101–17.
17. Liberati A, Altman DG, Tetzlaff J, Mulrow C, Gøtzsche PC, Ioannidis JPA, et al. The PRISMA statement for reporting systematic reviews and meta-analyses of studies that evaluate health care interventions: explanation and elaboration. PLoS Med. 2009;6(7):e1000100.
18. Willis BH, Quigley M. The assessment of the quality of reporting of meta-analyses in diagnostic research: a systematic review. BMC Med Res Methodol. 2011;11:163.
19. Greco T, Zangrillo A, Biondi-Zoccai G, Landoni G. Meta-analysis: pitfalls and hints. Heart Lung Vessels. 2013;5(4):219–25.

2 Diagnostic Studies Made Easy

Fikri M. Abu-Zidan, Marco Ceresoli, and Saleh Abdel-Kader

2.1 Introduction

Diagnostic methods are one of the major pillars of our daily surgical practice. We routinely encounter a young lady who visits the clinic because she has noticed a breast mass and she is worried that it is malignant, or an elderly man who noticed a change in his bowel habit associated with bleeding per rectum and he is worried that he has colonic malignancy. Alternatively, we may admit a boy to the hospital with suspected appendicitis and we need to decide whether to operate on him or not. To properly solve these problems and to answer patients' concerns, we routinely use diagnostic studies to help us. Whether these methods are radiological, laboratory, endoscopic, or interventional, the main objective of these studies is to guide our clinical decision in finding whether the patient has that suspected disease or not, or occasionally to predict their clinical outcome. Understandably, the benefit of these diagnostic studies should overweigh their side effects especially for invasive procedures. The results of a diagnostic test can be dichotomous (either negative or positive, for example, a SARS-CoV2 PCR test), categorical (like the type of the breast tumor), ordinal (like staging), or continuous values (like the C-reactive protein level). These types of data are explained in more detail in Chap. 13. We aim to lay

F. M. Abu-Zidan (✉)
The Research Office, College of Medicine and Health Sciences, United Arab Emirates University, Al-Ain, United Arab Emirates

M. Ceresoli
General and Emergency Surgery Department, School of Medicine and Surgery, Milano-Bicocca University, Monza, Italy

S. Abdel-Kader
Department of Surgery, Ain Shams University, Cairo, Egypt

M. Ceresoli et al. (eds.), *Statistics and Research Methods for Acute Care and General Surgeons*, Hot Topics in Acute Care Surgery and Trauma,
https://doi.org/10.1007/978-3-031-13818-8_2

the principles of using these diagnostic tests in our clinical practice. This will help to critically appraise a diagnostic study, to design a diagnostic study, and to analyze its data.

Learning Objectives

- Understand the basic components of a diagnostic study.
- Recognize the criteria of a good diagnostic test.
- Define the predictor and outcome of a diagnostic study.
- Understand and be able to calculate the sensitivity, specificity, and predictive values of a test.
- Appreciate the importance of predictive values and likelihood ratios in clinical practice.
- Comprehend that the prior priority of a disease affects both the results and application of a diagnostic test.
- Highlight the most common mistakes encountered in submitted diagnostic study articles.

2.2 Nature of a Diagnostic Study

In principle, diagnostic studies are similar to the observational studies. Nevertheless, observational studies are usually designed to investigate the epidemiology of a disease, explore its etiology, or define its outcome. In contrast, diagnostic studies are commonly designed to answer the question whether the patient has a disease or not.

2.3 The Need for a Gold Standard

How can we reach the disease real status? It can only be reached by using a **gold standard** having a definitive outcome. Ideally the gold standard should be positive in almost all patients with the disease and negative in almost all patients without the disease. This may be an excisional biopsy of a breast mass or an appendectomy with proven histopathology for positive cases. Is this the same for negative cases? Definitely not. We will not operate on negative cases to prove that they were negative but we reach that conclusion mainly with follow-up of the patients. It sometimes gets a little tricky. Let us say that we want to study the diagnostic ability of ultrasound in detecting free intraperitoneal fluid in blunt abdominal trauma. We may decide to consider CT scan as our gold standard although it is not perfect. Occasionally, we may consider the gold standard as CT scan or laparotomy because laparotomy is more accurate than the CT scan. The gold standard is usually used to rule in the disease than to rule it out. The definition of the disease outcome based on a selected gold standard is the most important pillar of a successful diagnostic study.

2.4 Components of Diagnostic Studies

Let us consider the scenario of a male patient presenting with pain in the right iliac fossa. Once you examined his abdomen, you found that it was tender but soft. You are not sure clinically whether the patient has appendicitis or not, so you decided to perform an abdominal CT scan with intravenous contrast to help you in your surgical decision. The result of the CT scan (*test result* whether diagnostic of appendicitis or not) is the *predictor*, and your *outcome* is the disease (whether present or absent). You may decide to observe the patient or operate on him depending on the result. If you have already decided to operate before performing the study, then there is no value of performing the study. This actually may delay your management.

Let us say that the CT scan result showed acute appendicitis (positive result) and then you operated on the patient, removed the appendix, and sent it for histopathology. The appendix can be inflamed (true positive) or normal (false positive). Conversely, the CT scan was normal and you decided to observe the patient. The patient may improve so the result of the CT scan is true negative. In comparison, the patient may develop a frank picture of localized peritonitis and once you operate on the patient, he had an acute perforated appendicitis. Then the result of the CT scan is false negative. This is demonstrated in Fig. 2.1.

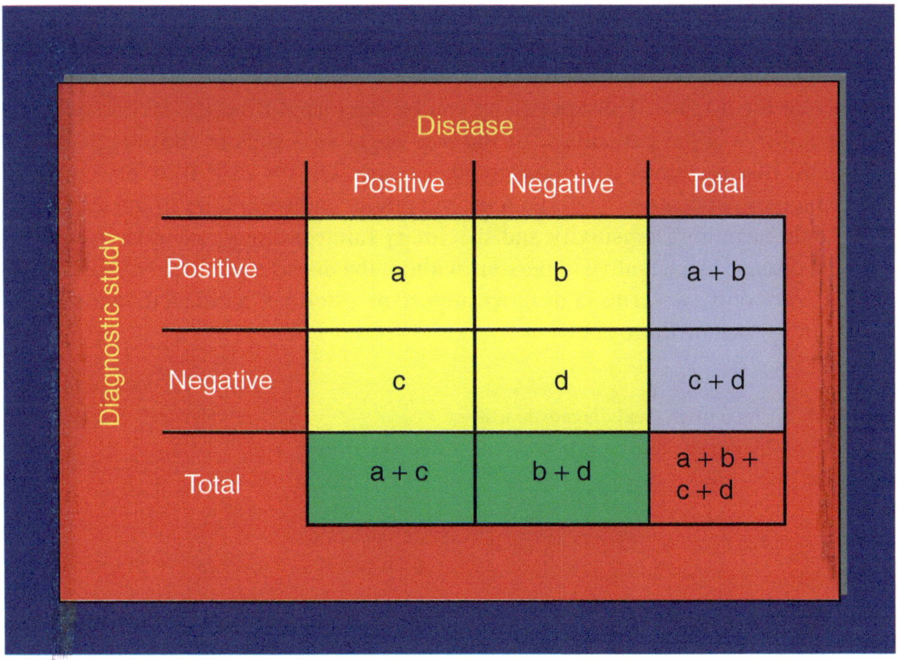

Diagnostic study	Disease: Positive	Disease: Negative	Total
Positive	a	b	a + b
Negative	c	d	c + d
Total	a + c	b + d	a + b + c + d

Fig. 2.1 A diagram showing the four cells stemming from the possibilities of the diagnostic study results depending on the disease status of the patient. *a* = true positive result (TP), *b* = false positive result (FP), *c* = false negative result (FN), and *d* = true negative result (TN)

Let us look at Fig. 2.1 carefully and take some time to digest it. That is the key for understanding, designing, and analyzing a diagnostic study. The real disease status is presented by the columns whether it is positive or negative. The results of the test are presented by the rows. Again, it is important to have this mental picture, status of the disease is in the vertical columns, while the results of the diagnostic study are in the horizontal rows. Just to simplify the idea, we will use the term normal for those who do not have the specific disease (although they may have another pathology). Accordingly, we will have four cells: (1) a cell for the positive tests in the diseased patients (a) which are the true positive (TP) results; (2) a cell for the positive tests in the normal patients (b) which are the false positive (FP) results; (3) a cell for the negative tests in the diseased patients (c) which are the false negative (FN) results; and (4) a cell for the negative tests in the normal patients (a) which are the true negative (TN) results.

The next step is to add the cells of each column and each row to have their total. This will give the number of real diseased patients ($a + c$), the number of normal patients ($b + d$); the total number of positive studies ($a + b$), the total number of negative studies ($c + d$), and the total number (n) of study population ($a + b + c + d$).

The third step is to pause, think, and look into the table again. This table can give us two important sides of the diagnostic study: the test and the patient. There are two important criteria that are related to the test which are sensitivity and specificity. Test **sensitivity** measures the ability of a test to detect presence of the disease. It can be calculated from the first column. It is the percentage of the true positive results in those having the disease. This can be calculated by $a/a + c$, in other words TP/TP + FN. In contrast, test **specificity** measures the ability of a test to detect the absence of the disease. This specificity can be calculated from the second column. The specificity is the percentage of the true negative results in those patients not having the disease which is $d/b + d$, in other words TN/TN + FP. It is very common that clinicians concentrate mainly on the sensitivity and specificity of a test. A good test should have high sensitivity and specificity (almost always positive in persons with the disease and negative in persons without the disease, preferably above 90%) but these are only two criteria of other important criteria of an ideal diagnostic test which are shown in Table 2.1.

Table 2.1 Criteria of an ideal diagnostic test

Criteria
Accurate
Simple
Safe
Non-expensive
Non-invasive
Fast
Painless
Has point-of-care option
Reliable
Easy to learn
Generalizable

2.5 Predictive Values

Kindly note that we have looked only at one side of a diagnostic study which is the test. But that is not the way we clinically practice surgery. Figure 2.2 shows the normal process of using a diagnostic test in our practice. Once we meet a patient with a specific complaint, we listen to him/her, examine the patient, decide whether we need a diagnostic test, ask for one if deemed necessary, wait for the results, and finally get the results. The result can be conclusive being positive or negative or may not even give an answer (non-conclusive). In that case, we may need to select another test which can give the answer.

The clinical reality is that a clinician gets a test result (positive or negative) and ponders how accurate this result is in predicting the real disease status of the patient. These are actually the predictive value of a positive test and the predictive value of a negative test. These can be calculated from the horizontal rows (Fig. 2.1).

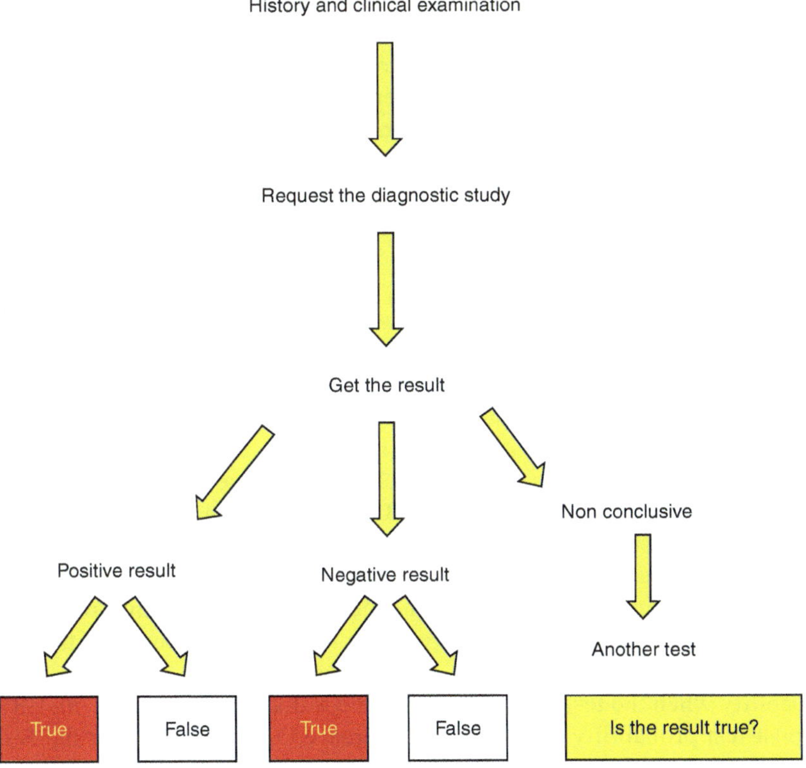

Fig. 2.2 A diagram demonstrating the natural process of the encounter between the doctor and the patient and the usual process for requesting a diagnostic study

The predictive value of a positive test in a study is the probability that a patient with a positive result actually has the disease. This can be calculated from the first row of Fig. 2.1 which is *a*/*a* + *b*, in other words TP/TP + FP. **The predictive value of a negative test** in a study is the probability that a patient with a negative result actually does not have the disease. This can be calculated from the second row of Fig. 2.1 which is *d*/*c* + *d*, in other words TN/TN + FN. Just to remember, if you evaluate the sensitivity or specificity of a test, calculate vertically. If you evaluate the predictive value of a positive or a negative result, calculate horizontally. Remember that we read horizontally not vertically, and attach that mentally to the clinical importance of the predictive values which is more important than the sensitivity and specificity.

2.6 Prior Probability of the Disease (Prevalence)

There is a need to define the prior probability of the disease in the studied population because the predictive values and the clinical implications of the test when using the likelihood ratios in decision-making will differ depending on the prior probability of the disease. The predictive value of a positive test (PPV) will increase with the increased prior probability. The prior probability of the disease (prevalence) is defined as the percentage of patients who have the disease out of those tested for the disease. In other words, TP + FN/total number of patients (*n*).

2.7 The Likelihood Ratio (LR)

It is the likelihood that a patient having the disease would have a certain test result divided by the likelihood that a patient without the disease would have the same result. In other words, it is the ratio of the true positive rate to the false positive rate. Sensitivity is the true positive rate, while 1 − specificity is the false positive rate. Accordingly, LR can be calculated as sensitivity/(1 − specificity).

The likelihood ratio is very useful in clinical practice when it is high because of its discriminating power. Figure 2.3 shows the Fagan nomogram. It is a graph which is used to estimate the extent of change in the probability that a patient has a disease depending on the likelihood ratio. The figure gives a theoretical comparison between two diagnostic tests (A and B) that were used to diagnose the disease in the same population having a prevalence of the disease (pre-test probability) of 50%. The diagram enabled us to define the post-test probability when the test was positive. In the A diagnostic test, having LR of 5, the post-test probability of the disease increased to 82% while for the B diagnostic test having LR of 1 the post-test probability of the disease stayed the same at 50%.

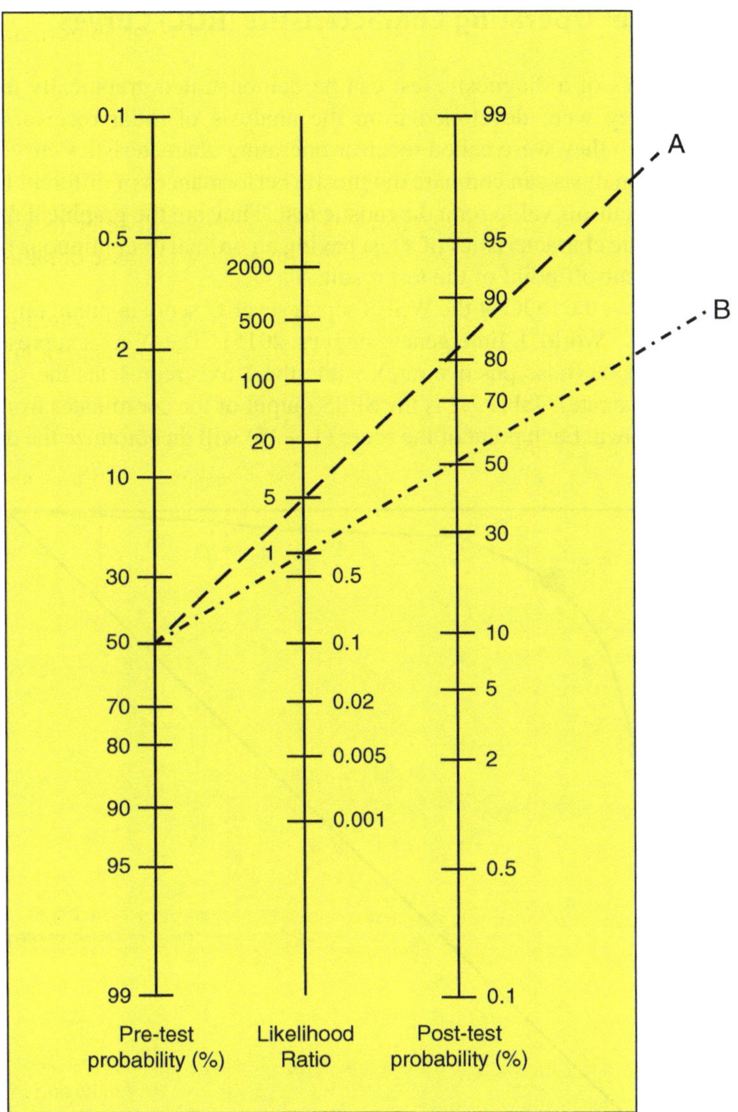

Fig. 2.3 A Fagan nomogram is used to estimate the extent of change of the probability that a patient has a disease depending on the likelihood ratio. The figure compares two diagnostic tests (A and B) that were used to diagnose the disease in the same population having a prevalence of the disease of 50%. For the A diagnostic test, having LR of 5, the post-test probability of the disease increased to 82% while for the B diagnostic test having LR of 1 the post-test probability of the disease stayed the same at 50%

2.8 Receiver Operating Characteristics (ROC) Curves

The characteristics of a diagnostic test can be demonstrated graphically using the ROC curves. They were developed from the analysis of radar receivers during WWII from which they were called receiver operating characteristics curves. ROC curves and their analysis can compare diagnostic performances of different tests and evaluate the best cut-off value for a diagnostic test. They are the graphical representation of diagnostic characteristics of a test having an ordinal or continuous outcome at each possible cut-off point of the test result.

Figure 2.4 shows the ROC of the WSES sepsis severity score in predicting mortality (Sartelli et al., World J Emergency surgery 2015). The *X* axis represents the 1 – Specificity value (false positive rate), while the *Y* axis represents the sensitivity value (true positive rate). Table 2.2 is the SPSS output of the coordinates from which this graph was drawn. Each point of the score (1 – 15) will dichotomize the data. The

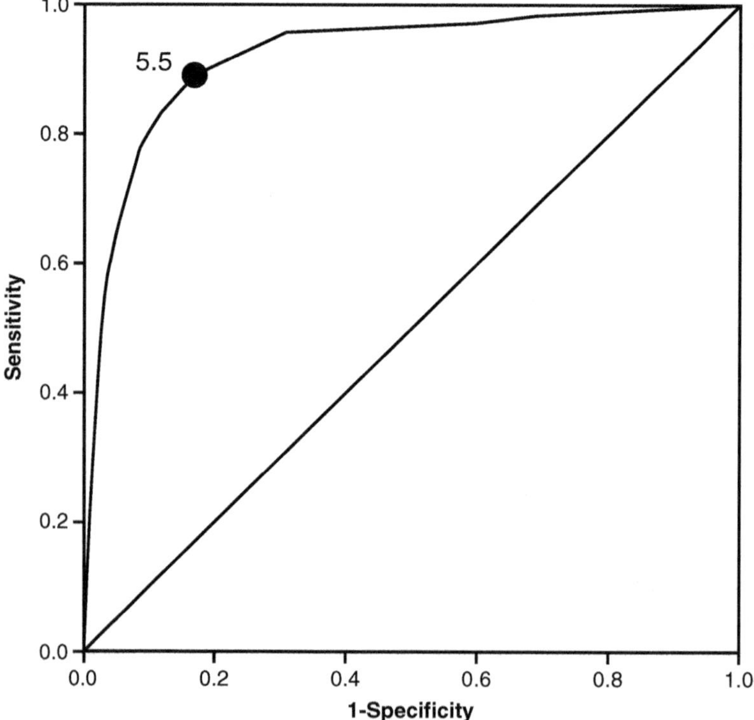

Fig. 2.4 Receiver operating characteristics (ROC) curve for the best WSES sepsis severity score that predicted mortality in patients having complicated intra-abdominal infection, global study of 132 centers ($n = 4553$). The best cut-off point for predicting mortality was 5.5. (Reproduced from the study of Sartelli M et al. Global validation of the WSES Sepsis Severity Score for patients with complicated intra-abdominal infections: a prospective multicenter study (WISS Study). World J Emerg Surg 2015; 10: 61 which is distributed under the terms of the Creative Commons Attribution 4.0 International License)

Table 2.2 SPSS outcome for the WSES sepsis severity score study with the coordinates of the data which were used to produce the ROC so as to define the best cut-off point of the score that predicts death

Positive if more than or equal to	Sensitivity	1 − Specificity
−1	1	1
0.5	0.986	0.766
1.5	0.986	0.725
2.5	0.978	0.653
3.5	0.964	0.395
4.5	0.942	0.323
5.5	**0.896**	**0.221**
6.5	0.802	0.101
7.5	0.757	0.081
8.5	0.598	0.043
9.5	0.436	0.019
10.5	0.335	0.013
11.5	0.159	0.004
12.5	0.101	0.001
13.5	0.024	0
15	0	0

Note that 5.5 had the best sensitivity and specificity

test will be considered true positive if death occurred at the WSES severity score which is greater than or equal to that point. It will be considered true negative if survival occurred if the score was less than that point. The test will be considered false positive if survival occurred at a score which is greater than or equal to that point and will be considered false negative if death occurred at a score less than that point. These dots draw a curve that describes the diagnostic accuracy of the WSES sepsis severity score in predicting mortality. A perfect test is the one which can vertically reach the left upper corner and then becomes horizontal. This would have a sensitivity of 100% and specificity of 100%. The diagonal line represents the reference line and is the result of a test that has 50% of specificity and 50% of sensitivity (like a coin tossing). The best cut-off point is usually where the curve turns with a corner, which was 5.5 in this case.

Another important element of the graph is the area depicted by the curve, called area under the curve (AUC): the higher this value, the higher is the diagnostic accuracy. The area under the reference line is 0.5 and represents a test with no diagnostic abilities. A test with good sensitivity and specificity will have a higher AUC: the maximum is 1. The AUC of the WSES sepsis severity score in predicting mortality was 0.92.

Let us take our trauma registry as another example. We want to evaluate the diagnostic performances of age and injury severity score (ISS) in predicting mortality of trauma patients. Figure 2.5 shows the diagnostic performances of age (blue line) and ISS (green line) in predicting trauma death. The AUC of age was 0.687 and the AUC of ISS was 0.92. ISS shows a better diagnostic performance in predicting mortality with a higher AUC compared with age.

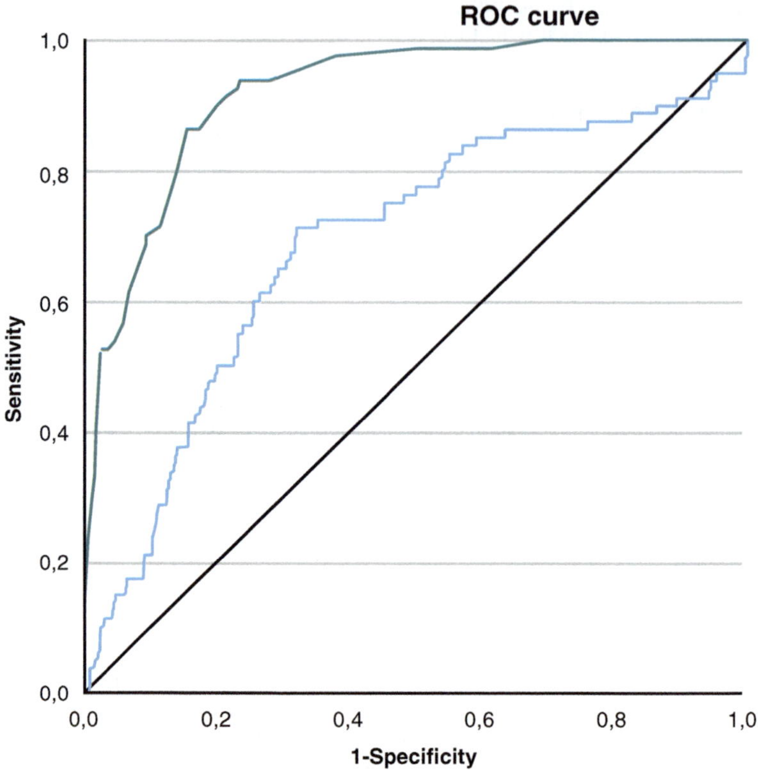

Fig. 2.5 Receiver operating characteristic (ROC) curve comparing the ability of age (blue line) and ISS (green line) in predicting trauma mortality. The area under the curve (AUC) of age was 0.687 and of ISS was 0.92 indicating that ISS had a much better predictor ability

2.8.1 Choosing a Cut-off Point: The Youden Index

What cut-off value can we choose to predict mortality in our clinical practice? According to the cut-off point chosen, the test will have different diagnostic abilities. A high cut-off point will produce a very specific test (low false positive rate because patients having an ISS above the chosen cut-off point will have a very high probability of death) but also a low sensitive test (high false negative rate because mortality may occur with ISS less than the chosen cut-off point).

On the contrary if we choose a low cut-off point we will have a very sensitive test (low false negative rate because death is unlikely if the ISS is less than the chosen cut-off point) but a poorly specific test (high false positive rate). Choosing the best cut-off point of a diagnostic test is not straightforward and should take into consideration the clinical contest. For example, some diseases require high sensitivity (screening tests) and others require high specificity. It is clear that the cut-off point plays a pivotal role in balancing diagnostic characteristic of a test (sensitivity and specificity).

To evaluate the best cut-off point, we can adopt the Youden's J statistics of Youden's index. For each cut-off point we can calculate the Youden's index as *"Sen sitivity + Specificity − 1."* This index could assume values between 0 and 1, where value 1 indicates the perfect diagnostic test. The cut-off value with the highest Youden's index indicates the value with the maximum available sensitivity and specificity.

2.9 Common Errors Encountered in Submitted Diagnostic Studies

We hope that by highlighting common errors of diagnostic studies, we will educate young researchers to avoid them when submitting their articles to journals. This will possibly reduce the chance of rejection of their papers. Other common errors encountered in research design are detailed in Chap. 3. Those that we have encountered when reviewing diagnostic studies submitted to acute care surgical journals include:

1. *No clear gold standard*: Using a gold standard is pivotal to assure the validity of the study. Missing the gold standard indicates that you cannot be sure of your results.
2. *Lack of definition of the test results:* The definition of each of the results (true positive, true negative, false positive, and false negative) should be clearly defined in the protocol and should be followed through the whole study.
3. *Not reporting the predictive values or likelihood ratio*: These important clinical values should be calculated and reported. Reporting only sensitivity and specificity is not enough.
4. *Ignoring the learning curve of the operator:* This is a common problem in diagnostic tests that need high technical skills. If the results of the study depend on the skill of the operator like laparoscopy or ultrasound, then the operator should have passed the learning curve stage so the poor results of the test are not attributed to the operator.
5. *Improper study population*: This can be a fatal mistake. The studied population should be that which will benefit from the study. An example for that is selecting a population that has a very high prior probability of the disease like studying the role of C-reactive protein in diagnosing acute appendicitis in those who were already operated. Those who were operated will have a prior probability of almost 90% of acute appendicitis which may be even higher than the sensitivity of the diagnostic test.
6. *Not addressing the generalizability:* Diagnostic studies should be useful in the real clinical situation for a particular setting. For example, the excellent results of diagnosing acute appendicitis by ultrasound experts may not be reproducible in other hospitals without proper training or expertise.
7. *Ignoring the non-conclusive findings:* The percentage of the non-conclusive results should be reported because it may affect the practical usefulness of the test. It is very interesting to note that many diagnostic studies ignore the

non-conclusive studies. These should be minimum to have a test which is useful. Let us assume that a study was done in a population and it was not conclusive in 50% of the patients, do you consider this as a good test!

Do and Don't

- Think about the components of the diagnostic studies you use.
- Use the predictive values and likelihood ratios in your clinical practice.
- Value the impact of prior priority of the disease on the results of diagnostic studies.
- Understand the structure of a diagnostic study. This will help to avoid common errors encountered in designing diagnostic studies.
- Do not concentrate only on the sensitivity and specificity of a study and know their limitations.

Take Home Messages

- There are two major components of a diagnostic study: The method and the population in which it was used.
- Calculate the sensitivity and specificity vertically and calculate the predictive values of a test horizontally.
- Overusing unnecessary diagnostic methods can be sometimes misleading.

Conflict of Interest None declared by the author.

Further Reading

Boyko EJ. Ruling out or ruling in disease with the most sensitive or specific diagnostic test: short cut or wrong turn? Med Decis Mak. 1994;14:175–9.

Browner WS, Newman TB, Cummings SR. Designing a new study: III. Diagnostic tests. In: Hulley SB, Cummings SR, editors. Designing clinical trials. Baltimore: Williams and Wilkins; 1988. p. 87–97.

Clarke JR. A scientific approach to surgical reasoning. II. Probability revision-odds ratios, likelihood ratios, and bayes theorem. Theor Surg. 1990;5:206–10.

Clarke JR, Hayward CZ. A scientific approach to surgical reasoning. I. Diagnostic accuracy-sensitivity, specificity, prevalence, and predictive value. Theor Surg. 1990;5:129–32.

Clarke JR, O'Donnell TF Jr. A scientific approach to surgical reasoning. III. What is abnormal? Test results with continuous values and receiver operating characteristic (ROC) curves. Theor Surg. 1990;6:45–51.

Goldin J, Sayre W. A guide to clinical epidemiology for radiologists: part II statistical analysis. Clin Radiol. 1996;51:317–24.

Peacock JL, Peacock JL. Diagnostic studies. In: Peacock JL, Peacock JL, editors. Oxford handbook of medical statistics. 1st ed. Oxford: Oxford University Press; 2011. p. 339–51.

Common Pitfalls in Research Design and Its Reporting

3

Fikri M. Abu-Zidan

3.1 Introduction

Being involved in reviewing articles for high impact surgical journals for more than 25 years, I have repeatedly encountered certain errors in research methodology and statistical analysis regardless of the origin of the manuscripts, whether stemming from developed or developing countries. These errors can be easily avoided by asking for advice and proper planning. Some of these errors, although seem trivial, can be fatal because they cannot be saved retrospectively. Occasionally researchers may concentrate so much on the details, technicality, and complexity while missing the overall picture. That is similar to visualizing a sky tower or reading a chest X-ray. Details can be missed either because you are so far from it, or alternatively so close to it. Taking care of the overall aim and structure of a research project is as important as looking into the small details. This chapter aims to highlight some common research design and reporting errors, hoping that they will be avoided when performing a research project.

Learning Objectives

- Highlight the importance of properly defining a focused research question.
- Stress the importance of involving a research methodologist in the research project.

F. M. Abu-Zidan (✉)
The Research Office, College of Medicine and Health Sciences, United Arab Emirates University, Al-Ain, United Arab Emirates

M. Ceresoli et al. (eds.), *Statistics and Research Methods for Acute Care and General Surgeons*, Hot Topics in Acute Care Surgery and Trauma,
https://doi.org/10.1007/978-3-031-13818-8_3

- Recognize that fatal errors in research design include using invalid measurement tools and testing the wrong population.
- Recognize the difference between correlation and prediction.
- Understand the difference between clinical and statistical significance.
- Report the data properly and describe how to deal with missing data.

3.2 Unclear Research Question

The main research question is "What do you want to find in your study?" If this question is not focused, it will be difficult to have a proper plan (map) to reach that aim. I think that a proper research question is the most important component for a research project. Let us give a practical example. We know that road traffic collisions cause death. We may ask ourselves what causes this death. This may be caused by speed, slipping of a car in a rainy weather, distraction of the driver when using a cell phone, or not using a seatbelt. Real life situations are complex, and we will not be able to answer all these questions at the same time in a single study. You have to define exactly what you want to study. Selecting a wrong research question makes the whole study flawed. This is similar to horse racing in which the eyes of the horse are covered by eye blinkers so the horse can go only in one direction (forward) to win the race (Fig. 3.1). If the blinkers are removed, the horse will look around and slow down. Accordingly, the researcher should spend significant time to define the aim of the study and concentrate on answering it. After reaching the first aim, then the researcher can remove the eye blinkers, look around, and think of his/her next target, and so on. Each question will generate multiple new questions. It is then the duty of a good researcher to define the next important, relevant, and feasible question to answer. I personally aim at answering one question in each study. I discourage my research students to have a multifactorial design in which they try to answer more than one question because this approach has the risk of not being able to

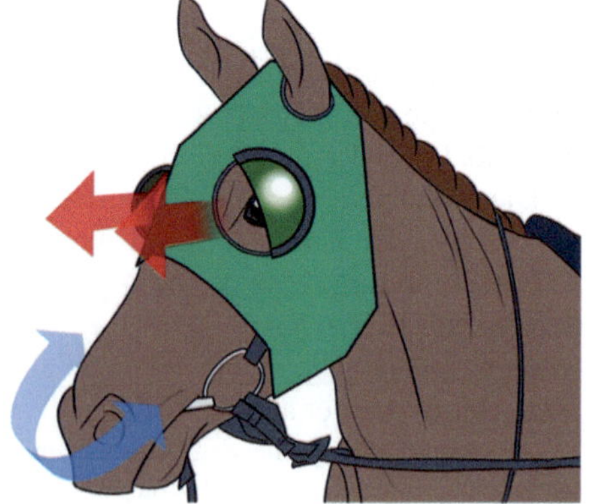

Fig. 3.1 Researchers should be like racing horses in their research in which the eyes of horses are covered by eye blinkers so that they can follow the racing track in one direction (forward) to win the race without being distracted. (*Illustrated by Mohammad F. Abu-Zidan*)

answer any of the questions. That is logical because having multiple questions to answer at the same time needs extreme care in the methods to be able to answer all questions. Making the aim more focused makes the methods simpler, direct, and more precise.

3.3 Lack of Planning *(Failing to Plan Is Planning to Fail)*

Genuine time should be spent in designing and planning a study before it starts. Involving a methodologist at this early stage will avoid errors and improve the chance of accepting a scientific paper. Submitted papers without involvement of a methodologist are more likely to be directly rejected without sending them to the reviewers. Even if they were sent for review, they are more likely to be rejected [1]. Inappropriate statistics and overinterpretation of the results are the most common causes for paper rejections [2]. Methodologists can be involved in the whole process of research including formulating the research question, research design, research audit, analyzing the data, participating in writing the manuscript, critically reading it, and finally approving it [3]. I will give a personal practical example highlighting this important point. Twenty years ago, I developed an experimental animal model for training Focused Assessment Sonography of Trauma (FAST) [4]. Designing and planning this study took 2 months, while performing the animal experiments and collecting the data took only 2 days. The paper was reviewed and accepted in less than 3 weeks. The ratio between the design/planning: performing the study in this example was 30:1. Although this may be an extreme example, it highlights the importance of thinking deeply and discussing the study with a methodologist to finalize the research design and plan for executing it.

3.4 Using the Wrong Research Tool

When measuring outcome variables in a research study, you need the proper tools to accurately measure these variables. Let us assume that you want to measure the mean arterial pressure in a critically ill septic patient in the intensive care unit. There are important characteristics in the measurement tool that have to be fulfilled. These are: (1) The tool should be *valid*, which means that it can measure the mean arterial pressure. Using a thermostat to measure the mean arterial pressure is not valid; (2) It should be *accurate*, this means that it will measure the real value; (3) It should be reliable, this means that it will give the same result if the measurements are repeated. Kindly note that accuracy is different from reliability. You may get the same result when the tool is reliable but this may cause a systematic error if it is not accurate. The most serious error in the study is using an invalid tool. This error cannot be corrected after finishing the study or experiment and will spoil the whole experiment.

It is common that acute care surgeons use surveys in their research. Although surveys look easy to perform and collect information about needs assessment, they are very tricky. They are not simply sending few questions and collecting the answers. It is important that these surveys should be valid and reliable. A lot of attention should be taken to have simple, clear, useful, well understood, and precise questions in these questionnaires [5].

3.5 Selecting the Wrong Population

This is a very fatal mistake that should be avoided. Any experiment or intervention should be tested in the population that are expected to benefit from it. I have repeatedly encountered clinical studies that aim to investigate a diagnostic test for a certain disease and then studied it in a population that has the final diagnosis of that disease (prior probability of almost 100%). An example of that is studying the role of ultrasound in diagnosing acute appendicitis. The authors studied ultrasound only in those operated (prior probability of 90%). That is the wrong population to be studied because ultrasound should be tested in those suspected to have appendicitis and not those already decided to be operated on. What is the value of ultrasound if you have already decided for surgery?

Let us have another example of an interventional procedure. Assume that we are going to study the role of Resuscitative Endovascular Balloon Occlusion of the Aorta (REBOA) in trauma abdominal bleeding patients. Figure 3.2 shows what is called the therapeutic window of an intervention. If REBOA was used in those having very mild disease, then it will be harmful (line is horizontal, no benefit). Similarly, if severity is above a certain limit (the line is also horizontal with severe injury), then it may not be useful. It is then very important to carefully select the population that may benefit from an intervention to be properly tested.

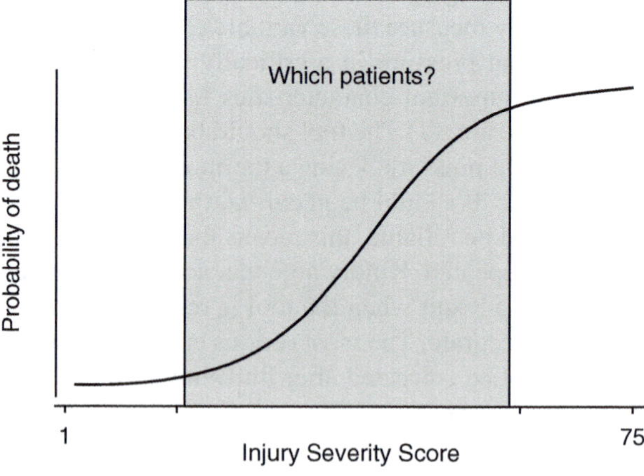

Fig. 3.2 An illustration showing the principle of the therapeutic window when using Resuscitative Endovascular Balloon Occlusion of the Aorta (REBOA). REBOA will be harmful if used in mild injured patients (lower horizonal line). It will not be useful if used above a certain limit (upper horizontal line)

3.6 Addressing the Missing Data

The authors have to be transparent regarding handling their missing data [3]. Prospective studies should generally have missing data of less than 10%. Retrospective studies usually have more missing data (up to 30%). Missing data are usually not random in high risk situations (like death) and may affect the analysis. Patients who die especially in the Emergency Department tend to have more missing data.

If imputations are used to replace the missing data (usually for retrospectively collected data), the authors have to justify this approach and demonstrate that missing data were random. This can be addressed by demonstrating that: (1) the groups have the same percentage of missing data before imputation for each studied variable and (2) they were statistically similar before the imputation. Our Trauma Group follows a school that does not replace missing data because this depends on assumptions which may increase the uncertainty in our statistical findings. We found that the best approach in establishing our trauma registry is to collect data prospectively by trained researchers and regularly audit the data which increased the trust in our data [6, 7].

3.7 Correlation and Prediction

There is great difference between correlation and prediction which should be clear. Correlation addresses the relationship between two variables regardless of whether one of them depends on the other. The correlation (association) does not imply a cause–effect relationship or the sequence in which they happen [8]. In comparison, prediction tries to define the outcome of one variable (dependent factor) depending on one or more factors (independent factors). The size of the p value does not reflect the strength of the correlation. Statistical significance having a small p value can occur when the sample size is large despite a weak correlation [9, 10]. Although there may be a statistically significant correlation, this may not be a strong correlation and the variable cannot be used as a predictor (Fig. 3.3). Predictors for important clinical outcomes, which can affect serious decisions, should be strong and simple to be useful in clinical practice.

The test for defining the correlation depends on whether the data have a normal distribution or not. When the data have a normal distribution, then Pearson's correlation test can be done. If the data are ordinal or do not have a normal distribution then Spearman's rank correlation test should be performed [8]. Figure 3.4 demonstrates this point. Spearman's rank correlation was used because the Likert type scale has ordinal data of 1–7. This analysis correlates the ranks and not the actual numbers. The scatterplot clearly shows that Pearson's correlation cannot be used in this scenario.

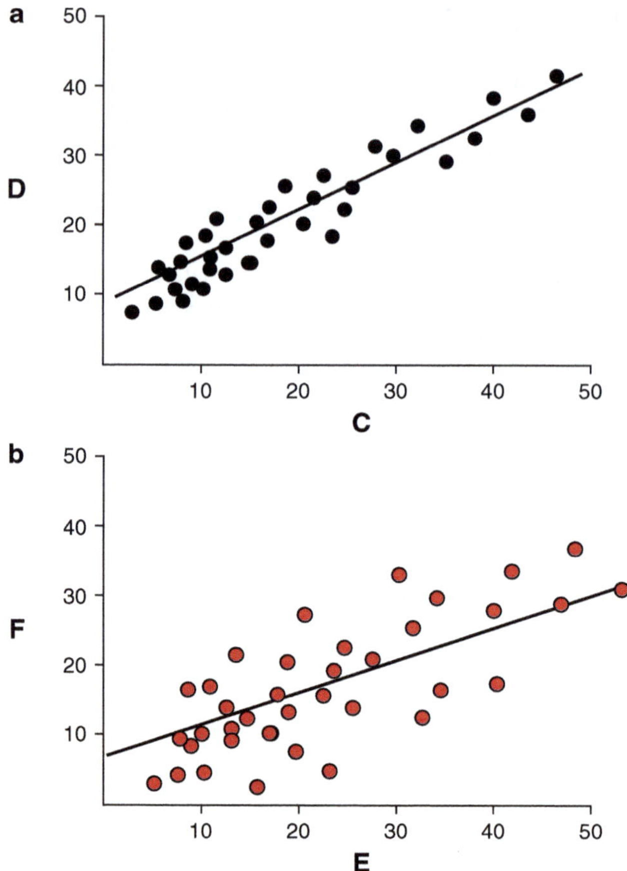

Fig. 3.3 This figure illustrates two situations of significant correlations; one of them has a strong correlation (**a**) that may be used for prediction, while the other has a weak correlation (**b**). Kindly notice the distribution of the data points around the correlation line and the slope of the line in each situation. Statistical significance with a small *p* value can occur despite a weak correlation

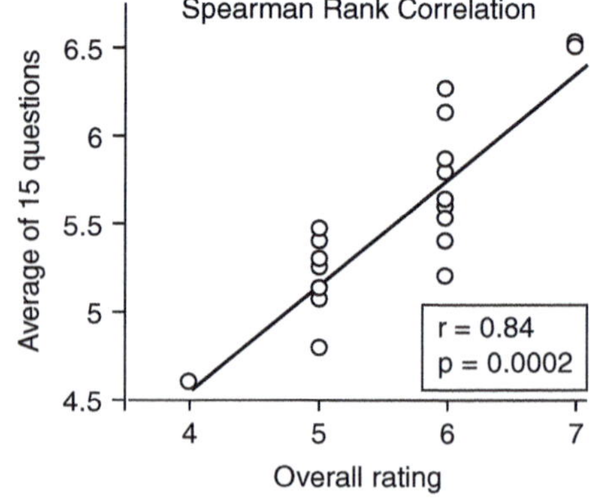

Fig. 3.4 The shown figure of the data of a Likert type scale has ordinal data of 1–7. The scatterplot clearly shows that Pearson's correlation cannot be used in this scenario. Spearman's rank correlation test should be used because the data do not have a normal distribution. This test correlates the ranks and not the actual numbers

3.7.1 Statistical and Clinical Significance

It is very important to be aware of the difference between statistical and clinical significance. We should not look through the pinhole of the *p* value but concentrate on the clinical implications of the statistical findings (Fig. 3.5). The "*p*" value estimates the probability that the reported result occurred by chance. It does not show the difference in the mean nor its direction. In contrast, confidence intervals can show the effect size, the direction of the change, the precision of the findings besides the statistical significance [11, 12].

Although statisticians can perform advanced analysis, clinicians may have more in-depth understanding of what do the findings mean because they are aware of their clinical importance and implications. Clinical significance depends on its effect on the existing clinical practice. When the sample size is large, there may be highly statistically significant findings but these may not translate to an effect size that can change clinical practice [13]. Occasionally when statisticians lead the clinical research, they may not appreciate the difference between dependent and independent factors if they do not have a clinical background or have close interactions with clinicians. I have personally reviewed articles in which the analysis tried to predict a clinically independent factor from a dependent factor which should be the opposite. Statisticians and clinicians should work together as one team before starting the clinical studies in designing the research protocol, during the study, and after completion of the study up to its publication. Team work is very important for acute care surgery including its research.

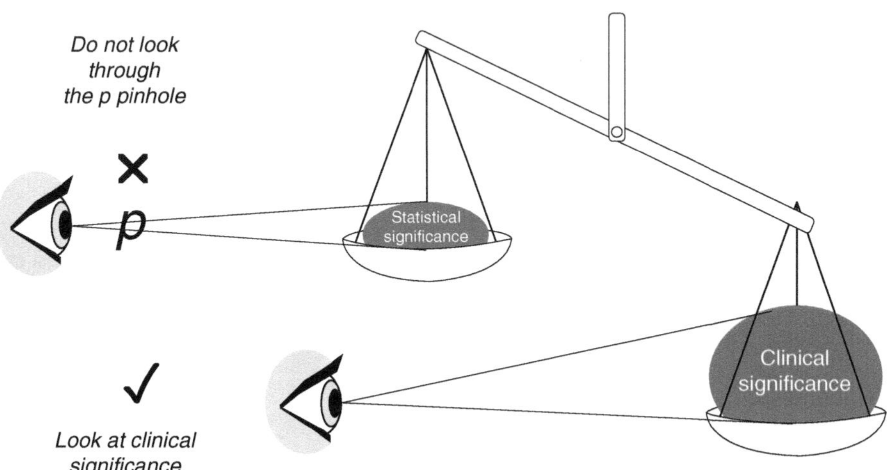

Fig. 3.5 We should not look through the pinhole of the "*p*" value but concentrate on the clinical implications of the statistical findings. The "*p*" value only estimates the probability that the reported result occurred by chance. It does not show the effect size nor its direction. (*Illustrated by Mohammad F. Abu-Zidan*)

3.8 Reporting of the Data

Accuracy and completion of the published statistical data will have long term implications in the future. Michalczyk and Lewis found that nearly half of the studies published in the Journal of Medical Education did not report enough statistical data [14]. Other researchers may need to compare the data with their own or pool the results in future systematic reviews. For example, it is not enough to report the mean alone without its variation (the standard deviation). In 2011, I had a disappointing personal experience trying to perform a systematic review on internal fixation of flail chest. After performing a lengthy detailed search, we could locate only two randomized controlled trials which were ready for the analysis [15, 16]. The paper of Granetzny et al. [15] reported only the mean without the standard deviation. We tried to contact the authors to get this data but we failed. Missing this simple data aborted the systematic review. When the mean and standard deviation of an independent variable of a group is given with the sample size, then it is possible to compare it or pool it with other studies [11]. It is becoming now a requirement in some highly ranked journals to publish the set of data that generated the results.

Do and Don't

- Define a focused, relevant, important, and feasible research question to answer.
- Plan your study properly with the help of a methodologist before you start data collection.
- Use valid tools to measure the outcome variables in the proper population.
- Report your data accurately.
- Concentrate on the clinical significance of your findings.
- Don't interpret a correlation relationship as a predictor.
- Don't ignore the missing data of your study.

Take Home Messages

- The research question is the most important pillar of a study.
- Failing to plan is planning to fail.
- Be transparent and accurate in using your research tools and reporting your results.
- Use your clinical sense.

Conflict of Interest None declared by the author.

References

1. Altman DG, Goodman SN, Schroter S. How statistical expertise is used in medical research. JAMA. 2002;287(21):2817–20.
2. Bordage G. Reasons reviewers reject and accept manuscripts: the strengths and weaknesses in medical education reports. Acad Med. 2001;76(9):889–96.

3. Clark GT, Mulligan R. Fifteen common mistakes encountered in clinical research. J Prosthodont Res. 2011;55(1):1–6.
4. Abu-Zidan FM, Siösteen AK, Wang J, Al-Ayoubi F, Lennquist S. Establishment of a teaching animal model for sonographic diagnosis of trauma. J Trauma. 2004;56:99–104.
5. Cummings SR, Hulley SB. Designing questionnaires and interviews. In: Hulley SB, Cummings SR, Browner WS, Grady DC, Newman TB, editors. Designing clinical research. 3rd ed. Philadelphia, PA: Lippincott Williams & Wilkins; 2007. p. 241–55.
6. Shaban S, Eid HO, Barka E, Abu-Zidan FM. Towards a national trauma registry for the United Arab Emirates. BMC Res Notes. 2010;3:187.
7. Shaban S, Ashour M, Bashir M, El-Ashaal Y, Branicki F, Abu-Zidan FM. The long term effects of early analysis of a trauma registry. World J Emerg Surg. 2009;4:42.
8. Chan YH. Biostatistics 104: correlational analysis. Singapore Med J. 2003;44:614–9.
9. Guyatt G, Walter S, Shannon H, Cook D, Jaeschke R, Heddle N. Basic statistics for clinicians: 4. Correlation and regression. CMAJ. 1995;152:497–504.
10. Aggarwal R, Ranganathan P. Common pitfalls in statistical analysis: the use of correlation techniques. Perspect Clin Res. 2016;7:187–90.
11. Bailar JC 3rd, Mosteller F. Guidelines for statistical reporting in articles for medical journals. Amplifications and explanations. Ann Intern Med. 1988;108:266–73.
12. Ranganathan P, Pramesh CS, Buyse M. Common pitfalls in statistical analysis: "P" values, statistical significance and confidence intervals. Perspect Clin Res. 2015;6:116–7.
13. Ranganathan P, Pramesh CS, Buyse M. Common pitfalls in statistical analysis: clinical versus statistical significance. Perspect Clin Res. 2015;6:169–70.
14. Michalczyk AE, Lewis LA. Significance alone is not enough. J Med Educ. 1980;55:834–8.
15. Granetzny A, Abd El-Aal M, Emam E, Shalaby A, Boseila A. Surgical versus conservative treatment of flail chest. Evaluation of the pulmonary status. Interact Cardiovasc Thorac Surg. 2005;4:583–7.
16. Tanaka H, Yukioka T, Yamaguti Y, Shimizu S, Goto H, Matsuda H, Shimazaki S. Surgical stabilization of internal pneumatic stabilization? A prospective randomized study of management of severe flail chest patients. J Trauma. 2002;52:727–32.

Part II

Basic Statistical Analysis

Introduction to Statistical Method

4

Luca Gianotti

4.1 Introduction

Medical statistics (or biostatistics) is fundamental for the study of human health and disease. Its applications range from biomedical laboratory research, to clinical medicine, to health promotion, to national and global systems of health care to medicine and the health sciences, including public health, forensic medicine, epidemiology, and clinical research. It is the science of summarizing, collecting, presenting, and interpreting data in medicine and using this data estimate the magnitude of associations and test hypotheses.

Two fundamental ideas in the field of statistics are uncertainty and variation. There are many situations that we encounter in science in which the outcome is uncertain. In some cases, the uncertainty is because the outcome in question is not determined yet, while in other cases the uncertainty is because although the outcome has been determined already we are not aware of it.

Probability is a mathematical language used to discuss uncertain events and probability plays a key role in statistics. Any measurement or data collection is subject to a number of sources of variation. It means that if the same measurements are repeated, then the answers would likely change. Statistics attempt to understand and control (where possible) the sources of variation in any situation and measure the probability.

L. Gianotti (✉)
School of Medicine and Surgery, Milano-Bicocca University, and HPB Unit, San Gerardo Hospital, Monza, Italy
e-mail: luca.gianotti@unimib.it

M. Ceresoli et al. (eds.), *Statistics and Research Methods for Acute Care and General Surgeons*, Hot Topics in Acute Care Surgery and Trauma,
https://doi.org/10.1007/978-3-031-13818-8_4

4.2 The Hypothesis

A scientific hypothesis is the initial building block in the scientific method. The basic idea of a hypothesis is that there is no pre-determined outcome. Thus, when a study or a protocol is designed, the hypothesis is your "best guess" about the effect of a treatment based on biological plausibility and previous literature results. A hypothesis can be formulated only in randomized controlled trials testing a treatment or in prospective observational studies challenging, for example, the prognostic or diagnostic ability of a test or a variable on a specified outcome.

Hypothesis testing requires the construction of a statistical model, meaning to test whether the data of an experiment follow a chance or casual processes or are truly responsible for the results obtained.

There are two types of hypothesis: the null hypothesis and the alternative hypothesis. The null hypothesis and the alternative hypothesis are types of conjectures used in statistical tests, which are formal methods of reaching conclusions or making decisions on the basis of data.

- The null hypothesis is the default hypothesis, also called zero hypothesis (H_0) because it implies that the difference to be measured is zero (null). It means that there is no difference between two or more observed measures or groups. Therefore, the main statistical assumption is the null hypothesis.
- The alternative hypothesis, also defined as H_1 hypothesis, is the opposite of the H_0 meaning that there is a significant difference between experimental groups or samples.

Very roughly, the procedure for deciding goes like this: Take a random sample from a population. If the sample data are consistent with the null hypothesis, then do not reject the null hypothesis; if the sample data are inconsistent with the null hypothesis, then reject the null hypothesis and conclude that the alternative hypothesis is true.

Example

Uncomplicated appendicitis may be treated conservatively with antibiotic therapy even though a 40% recurrence rate is described. A new antibiotic Z might reduce the probability of having an operation for uncomplicated appendicitis. Possible null hypotheses are "this antibiotic Z does not reduce the chances of having surgery" or "this antibiotic Z has no effect on the chances of having surgery." The test of the hypothesis consists of administering the new antibiotic Z to half of the population with uncomplicated appendicitis (study group) as compared to the other half of the population (control group) receiving antibiotic B which represents the standard of care. If the data show a statistically significant change in the people receiving antibiotic A, the null hypothesis is rejected and the H_1 hypothesis is accepted.

According to the study design with one, two, or more samples, comparing means, variances, or proportions, paired or unpaired data, with different distributions, or large and small sample size, there are many types of significance tests that can be used to test the hypotheses. The appropriate significant test to be used depends on the type of data you are handling.

As stated above a hypothesis may be formulated also in prospective observational studies.

Example

I wish to test if a certain level of C-reactive protein (CRP), measured at the first day after a major abdominal operation, is predictive of infectious complications occurring later on in the postoperative course. From literature review, but in a different population (cardiac surgery), the best threshold is > 5 mg/dL. A possible null hypothesis is "A CRP > 5 is not capable of predicting the occurrence of an infection." The test of the hypothesis consists of comparing the group of patients with CRP ≤ 5 with the group of patients with CRP > 5. If the data show a non-statistically different proportion of infections in the two groups, the null hypothesis is accepted.

4.3 The Aim

Much easier to apply and describe is the aim of a study that typically applies to retrospective research. Alternative terms for aim are goal, purpose, or objective of a study. As the hypothesis, the aim should be formulated based on "hole/s" in the previous knowledge of a research topic and put in the contest of the available literature. The aim/s should establish the scope, depth, and direction that a research will ultimately take. An effective set of aims will give the research focus and clarity for the readers. Therefore, the aims indicate what is to be achieved with the study and describe the main goal or the main purpose of the research project.

In doing so, it acts as a focal point for your research and should provide the readers with clarity as to what the study is all about. Because of this, research aims are almost always located within its own subsection under the introduction section of a research document.

A research aim is usually formulated as a broad statement of the main goal of the research and can range in length from a single sentence to a short paragraph. Although the exact format may vary according to preference, they should all describe why the research is needed (i.e. the context), and possibly what it sets out to accomplish.

Example

The use of preoperative biliary stenting (PBS) in jaundice patients with periampullary malignancy is debated. Current guidelines recommend to avoid routine biliary stenting and to limit the procedure to symptomatic jaundice, cholangitis, or planned neoadjuvant treatment. Despite delaying surgery by 4–6 weeks having been suggested, the time needed for recovery after biliary drainage is undefined, and no gold standard tests have been recognized to quantify the recovery of liver functions after PBS.

The aim of this study was to evaluate the potential association between the duration of PBS and the occurrence and severity of postoperative morbidity in patients undergoing pancreatoduodenectomy.

4.4 The Errors

A type I error [or alpha (α)] is a false positive conclusion, while a type II error [or beta (β)] is a false negative conclusion. Statistical planning always involves uncertainties, so the risks of making these errors are unavoidable in hypothesis testing. These risks can be minimized through careful planning in your study design. Using hypothesis testing, you can make decisions about whether your data support or refute your research predictions.

4.4.1 Type I Error

A type I error means rejecting the null hypothesis when it is actually true. It means concluding that results are statistically significant when, in reality, they came about purely by chance or because of unrelated factors.

The risk of committing this error is the significance level (or α) you choose. That is a value that you set at the beginning of your study to assess the statistical probability of obtaining your results (in other words, the *p* value). The significance level is usually set at 0.05 or 5%. This means that your results only have a 5% chance of occurring, or less, if the null hypothesis is actually true.

If the *p* value of your test is lower than the significance level, it means your results are statistically significant and consistent with the alternative hypothesis. If your *p* value is higher than the significance level, then your results are considered statistically non-significant.

Example

It is established that repeated episodes of postoperative hyperglycemia in non-diabetic subjects increase the risk of having surgery-related infections after major abdominal operations and it is also known that preoperative oral carbohydrate (CHO) loading blunts insulin resistance and thus decreases the risk of hyperglycemia. Therefore, you design a trial to explore whether preoperative oral CHO loading could achieve a reduction in the occurrence of postoperative infection when compared with the occurrence of postoperative infection with placebo. This calculated sample size equal to 440 patients per group is set to provide an 80% power (type II error) with a type I error rate fixed at 5% to detect superiority in a 40% reduction (effect size) of the rate of postoperative infection given an overall risk of infection equal to 18%. The results are as follows: Postoperative infections occurred

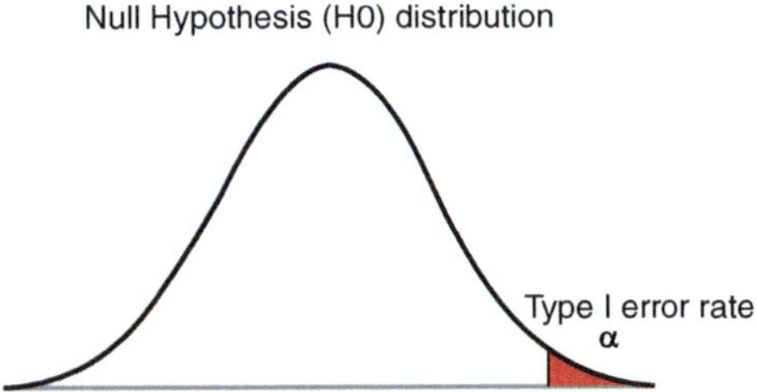

Fig. 4.1 The figure shows the distribution of the null hypothesis. If your results fall in the red area (alpha) there is a less than 5% of probability that the results are consistent with the null hypothesis

in 16.3% of patients from the CHO group and in the 16.0% patients from the placebo group (relative risk: 1.019, 95% confidential interval 0.720–1.442; relative difference 0.003, 95% confidential interval 0.053–0.059, P = 1.00).

In this case you are very confident in accepting the null hypothesis because the risk of a type I error is close to zero.

Let us hypothetically say that instead the results show that the CHO group has a rate of infections of 11.2% and in this case the p value is 0.04. Theoretically, you should reject the null hypothesis. However, this p value means that there is a 4% chance of your results occurring if the null hypothesis is true. Therefore, there is still a risk of making a type I error.

To reduce the probability of a type I error, you can simply set a lower significance level (i.e. 0.01).

4.4.2 Type I Error Rate

The null hypothesis distribution curve (shown below) displays the probabilities of obtaining all possible results if the study is repeated with new samples and the original null hypothesis holds true.

At the tail end, the shaded area represents alpha. If your results fall in this area of this curve, they are considered statistically significant and the null hypothesis is rejected (Fig. 4.1).

4.4.3 Type II Error

A type II error means not rejecting the null hypothesis when it is actually false. Thus, a type II error means failing to conclude there was an effect when there actually was. In reality, your study may not have had enough statistical power to detect an effect of a certain size. Statistical power is the extent to which a test can correctly detect a real effect when there is one. A power level of 80% or higher is usually considered acceptable.

The risk of a type II error is inversely related to the statistical power of a study. The higher the statistical power, the lower the probability of making a type II error.

Example

You may consider the same case used to elucidate type I error. You run a subset analysis of that trial results and the rate of infections in women (representing half of the entire population) is 15% in the placebo group vs. *11% in the CHO group with a p value of 0.08. Though, by analyzing this subgroup (women) you have reduced the sample size. In this case you should accept the null hypothesis and concluding that the CHO treatment does not affect the outcome even in this specific subgroup of subjects. However, this may represent a type II error and the effect of treatment is not significant only because you have reduced the sample. In other words, you are failing to conclude there is an effect when there actually is.*

A type II may occur if an effect is smaller than this size. A smaller effect size is unlikely to be detected in your study due to inadequate statistical power.

4.4.4 Statistical Power

The statistical power of a hypothesis test is the probability of detecting an effect if there is a true effect present to detect.

Statistical power is determined by:

- Effect size: Larger effects are more easily detected.
- Sample size: Larger samples reduce sampling error and increase power.
- Significance level: Increasing the significance level (alpha) increases power.

To (indirectly) reduce the risk of a type II error, you can increase the sample size or the significance level.

4.4.5 Type II Error Rate

The alternative hypothesis distribution curve (shown below) depicts the probabilities of obtaining all possible results if the study is repeated with new samples and the original alternative hypothesis holds true. Type II error rate (β) is represented by the blue area on the left side. The remaining area under the curve represents statistical power, which is 1—β.

Increasing the statistical power of your test directly decreases the risk of making a type II error (Fig. 4.2).

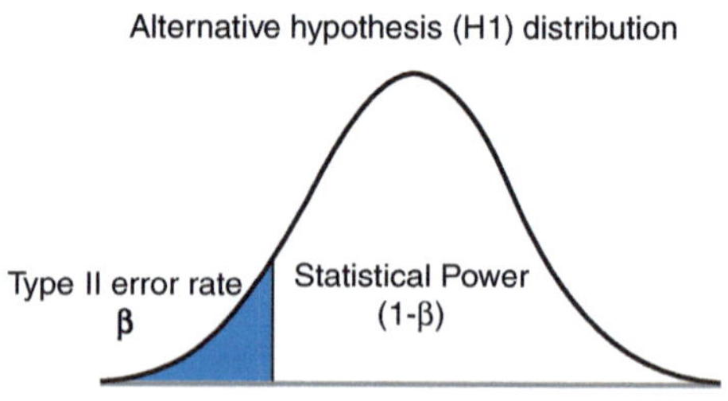

Fig. 4.2 The figure shows the distribution of the alternative H1 hypothesis. The blue area indicates type II error rate probability

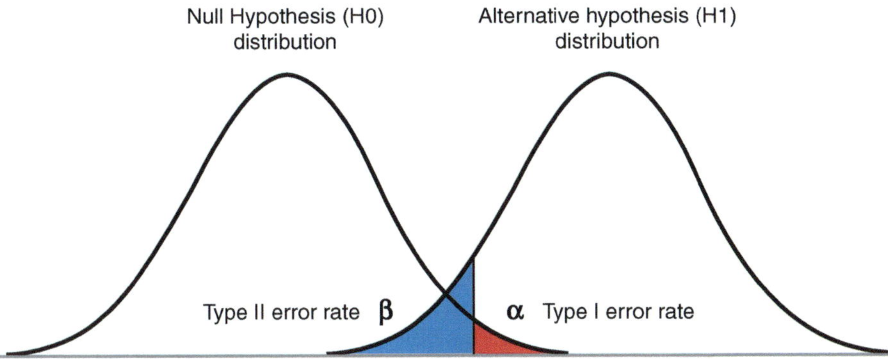

Fig. 4.3 The error trade-off. The distribution of the two hypothesis are always intersected

4.4.6 Trade-Off between Type I and Type II Errors

Type I and type II error rates influence each other. That is because the significance level (type I error rate) affects statistical power, which is inversely related to type II error rate.

This means there is an important trade-off between type I and II errors:

- Setting a lower significance level decreases a type I error risk, but increases a type II error risk.
- Increasing the power of a test decreases a type II error risk, but increases a type I error risk.

This trade-off is visualized in the graph below. Hypothesis distributions are not distant but are always intersected with an overlapping area. This overlapping area is the error area and it is divided into type I and type II errors. By setting type I error rate, you indirectly influence the size of type II error rate as well. Reducing the alpha always comes at the cost of increasing beta and vice versa (Fig. 4.3).

4.4.7 Is a Type I or Type II Error Worse?

There is no worse error, but both may have important consequences. A type I error means mistakenly going against the null hypothesis. This may lead to new policies, practices, or treatments that are inadequate or a waste of resources. In contrast, a type II error means failing to reject a null hypothesis. It may result in missed opportunities for new treatments or innovations.

4.5 Sample Size Calculation

One of the pivotal aspects of planning a clinical study is the calculation of the sample size. It is naturally neither practical nor feasible to study the whole population in any study. Hence, a set of participants is selected from the population, which is less in number (size) but adequately represents the population from which it is drawn so that true inferences about the population can be made from the results obtained. This set of individuals is known as the "sample."

In a statistical context the "population" is defined as the complete set of people (e.g. people of Italy with cholelithiasis). The "target population" is a subset of individuals with specific clinical and demographic characteristics in whom you want to study your intervention (e.g. symptomatic cholelithiasis), and "sample" is a further subset of the target population which we would like to include in the study (e.g. symptomatic cholelithiasis with signs of inflammation). Thus a "sample" is a portion, piece, or segment that is representative of a whole.

To calculate the sample of a study, four components are needed: type I error, type II error, the incidence of an event, and the relative variation. The calculation of the sample, from a mathematical and statistical point of view, will be not discussed in this chapter. However easy tool for sample size calculation is available online.

Examples
I want to study the effect in preventing wound infection of an antibiotic X versus *an antibiotic Z for preoperative prophylaxis in colorectal surgery.*

A. *I choose a type I error of 5% and a type II error of 80%, the recognized incidence of wound infection is 20%, and I expect a superior effect of antibiotic X with a relative reduction of incidence of 30% (absolute reduction to 14%). The sample size calculation is 1228 (614 for antibiotic X and 614 for antibiotic Z).*
B. *I choose a type I error of 1% and a type II error of 90%, the recognized incidence of wound infection is 20%, and I expect a superior effect of antibiotic X with a relative reduction of incidence of 30% (absolute reduction to 14%). The sample size calculation is 2328 (1164 for antibiotic X and 1164 for antibiotic Z).*
C. *I choose a type I error of 5% and a type II error of 80%, the recognized incidence of wound infection is 20%, and I expect a superior effect of antibiotic X with a relative reduction of incidence of 50% (absolute reduction to 10%). The sample size calculation is 398 (199 for antibiotic X and 199 for antibiotic Z).*

How do I decide on these 4 parameters? By convention it is acceptable to set a type I error at 5% (but not higher) and a type II error at 80% (but no lower). However, the value to attribute to the errors remains a free choice. The incidence of an event should be based on the existing literature or from previous observational study in your setting. The relative or absolute variation between study groups is your hypothesis and should be based on previous studies, biologic plausibility, or clinical relevance.

4.6 The *P* Value

The America Statistical Association (ASA) panel defined the *P* value as "the probability under a specified statistical model that a statistical summary of the data (for example, the mean or median difference between two compared groups) would be equal to or more extreme than its observed value" [1].

What does it mean for us (mortal human being) who read a scientific paper and want to get information on changing or not our routine clinical practice? It means that a *P* value ≤0.05 of any statistical test is not enough to accept or reject the null hypothesis. Therefore, part of the problem lies in how people interpret *P* values. According to the ASA statement, "A conclusion does not immediately become 'true' on one side and 'false' on the other." Valuable information may be lost because researchers may not pursue "insignificant" results. Conversely, small effects with "significant" *P* values may be biologically or clinically unimportant. At best, such practices may slow scientific progress and waste resources. At worst, they may cause harm when adverse effects go unreported or underestimated [2].

For a given dataset, researches can always find some group comparisons that eventually result in the magic number of *P* value ≤0.05 and then convince themselves that what turns to be "significant" is the key hypothesis and it has a lot of plausibility to the investigator.

How can we partially overcome the misinterpretation of the *P* value? For example, by looking at confidence intervals, effect sizes, or risks ratios which convey what a *P* value alone does not: the magnitude and relative importance of an effect.

Example

On April 26, 2021 it was published the largest randomized clinical trial comparing laparoscopic pancreatoduodenectomy (LPD) to open pancreatoduodenectomy (OPD) [3].

This trial was designed because the benefit and safety of LPD for the treatment of pancreatic or periampullary tumors remain controversial. Studies have shown that the learning curve plays an important role in LPD, yet there are no randomized studies on LPD after the surgeons have surmounted the learning curve. The aim of this trial was to compare the outcomes of OPD with those of LPD, when performed by experienced surgeons.

The researches set as primary endpoint of the trial the length of hospital stay assuming that LPD would confer benefit and thus reduce the duration of the hospitalization by almost 3 days. They calculated the sample size as follows: In a previous study, a mean reduction of 2.95 days was observed for patients undergoing LPD versus *OPD, with a standard deviation of 12.3 days. Assuming that the length of stay in the OPD group would be 12 days, for a two-sided test with a power (1–β) of 80% and a significance level (α) of 5%, the minimum number of patients required in each group was 274.*

4.6.1 Results and Interpretation

In the intention to treat statistical analysis, the median length of stay (Interquartile) was 15.0 (11.0–21.0) days for the LPD group versus 16.0 (13.0–21.0) days in the OPD with a difference of −1.8 day and relative 95% confidential interval of −3.3/0.3 and a *P* value of 0.02.

So, the *P* value was "significant" and a rushed interpretation should be: the laparoscopic procedure is better than the open procedure and therefore the null hypothesis is rejected. Is it really so? Is this a potential type I error? Is the *P* value alone reliable? If you look more deeply to the results, I may interpret this "significant" *P* value in a different way. First, the actual length of stay was higher than was postulated during the hypothesis generation. Second, the difference was smaller than what expected with a large confidential interval. Third and more important, is this difference so clinically important or for the patient well-being, or for the health care system?

Last but not least, let us have a look at additional results:

In the intention to treat statistical analysis the rate of major postoperative complications was 29% in the LPD versus 23% in the OPD group, with a risk ratio (95% confidential interval) of 1.23 (0.94–1.62) and a *P* value of 0.13. In the per-protocol analysis the rate of major complications was 30% in the LPD versus 21% in the OPD with a risk ratio of 1.42 (1.05–1.93) with a *P* value of 0.06. The comprehensive complication index (an overall measure of the burden of morbidly) followed the same trend.

So, the *P* value was "not significant" and a rushed interpretation should be: the laparoscopic procedure generates a similar risk of major postoperative complications than the open procedure and therefore the null hypothesis is accepted. Is it really so? How do I interpret the risk ratio? A risk ratio of 1.42 means that the LPD is associated with a 42% increased risk of having major complications when compared to OPD which although is "not significant" ($P = 0.06$). Is this a potential type II error? And more, is this difference (not statistically speaking) clinically important, or for the patient well-being, or for the health care system?

Last but not least, how I do interpret a significant reduction of the length of stay as opposite to a non-significant but substantial increase in major morbidity in the LPD groups?

The above is a reasonable example of how the results of the study may be misinterpreted by looking only at the *P* value.

4.7 Bias

A bias can be defined as "any process at any stage of inference which tends to produce results or conclusions that differ systematically from the truth" [4]. Therefore, a bias is a systematic error, or deviation from the truth, in results. Biases can lead to underestimation or overestimation of the true intervention effect. It is usually impossible to know to what extent biases have affected the results of a particular study or analysis. For these reasons, it is more appropriate to consider whether a result is at risk of bias rather than claiming with certainty that it is biased.

Bias should not be confused with imprecision. Bias refers to systematic error, meaning that multiple replications of the same study would reach the wrong answer on average. Imprecision refers to random error, meaning that multiple replications of the same study will produce different effect estimates because of sampling variation, but would give the right answer on average. Precision depends on the number of participants and the number of events in a study and is reflected in the confidence interval around the intervention effect estimate. The results of smaller studies are subject to greater sampling variation and hence are less precise. A small trial may be at low risk of bias yet its result may be estimated very imprecisely, due to a wide confidence interval. Conversely, the results of a large trial may be precise (narrow confidence interval) but also at a high risk of bias.

Bias should also not be confused with the external validity of a study, that is, the extent to which the results of a study can be generalized to other populations or settings. For example, a study may enroll participants who are not representative of the population who most commonly experience a particular clinical condition. The results of this study may have limited generalizability to the wider population, but will not necessarily give a biased estimate of the effect in the highly specific population on which it is based.

Biases can arise at three steps of the study: during initial enrollment of the participants, during implementation of the study, and during analysis of the findings.

The first source of bias arises from the absence of a control group in descriptive studies. Descriptive studies, such as cross-sectional studies and case series, select a group of patients based on a particular characteristic (e.g. a type of disease or treatment) and describe their evolution, for example, the disease course with a new treatment. Contrary to analytic studies, such, there is no control group for comparison. Thus, if a certain recovery rate is observed, it not only can be related to the treatment effect but also to several other parameters. For example, initial characteristics of the patients, natural evolution of the disease, placebo effect and, in the case of a comparison between pretreatment and post-treatment values, regression toward the mean could partially or totally explain the recovery.

Among analytic studies (such as case–control studies, cohorts, and randomized controlled trials) three major categories of bias can be recognized: selection bias, classification bias, and confounding bias.

4.7.1 Selection Bias

Selection bias occurs if the study population does not reflect a representative sample of the target population. Thus, the conclusion drawn by the study may not be extended to other patients. In randomized trials, proper randomization minimizes differential selection bias, although it is frequent in observational studies.

Example

I want to test whether oral antibiotics may avoid unnecessary surgery for Hinchey I stage diverticulitis and I compare patients under observation in hospital with a cohort of subjects that received the same antibiotics but they are suitable for home therapy. This is a clear selection bias since certain risk factors may be overrepresented in hospitalized subjects compared with the general population, and these risk factors may confound the findings independently of the disease in question.

In contrast, the following is not a selection bias. Let us imagine that I designed a RCT to compare two surgical techniques for elective laparoscopic cholecystectomy and some inclusion criteria are set: female patients with no comorbidities, BMI less than 25, and with less than 50 years of age. In this case the results cannot be simply generalized to the entire population with an indication to cholecystectomy.

Selection bias also can arise during implementation of the study. In observational studies, when losses or withdrawals are uneven in outcome categories. Such selection bias attributable to losses of follow-up is called attrition bias.

4.7.2 Classification Bias

Classification bias, also called measurement or information bias, results from improper, inadequate, or ambiguous recording of individual factors (either exposure or outcome variables). If the misclassifications occur randomly, the bias is said to be non-differential. On the contrary, if misclassifications are related to exposure, outcome, or treatment allocation, the classification bias is differential. In clinical trials, blinding prevents differential classification bias. Therefore, observational studies, and in particular, case–control retrospective studies are at major risk of classification bias. Classification bias also can occur if different methods of diagnosis are used for the patients.

Example

With a prospective observational study, I would like to find an association between preoperative muscle mass and risk of surgery-related morbidity after major oncologic operations. Muscle mass is measured in some patients by a CT-scan dedicated software, in others by bioimpedance analysis or dual-energy X-ray absorptiometry. The results of these three groups cannot be pulled if not at risk of manifest classification bias.

4.7.3 Confounding Bias

Confounding bias is a false association made between the outcome and a factor that is not itself causally related to the outcome and occurs if the factor is associated with a range of other characteristics that do increase the outcome risk. Thus, for a characteristic to be a confounder, it must be related to the outcome in terms of prognosis or susceptibility and be unequally distributed among the compared groups.

Confounding bias may mask an actual association or, more commonly, falsely demonstrate an apparent association between the treatment and outcome when no real association between them exists.

Example

I wish to study the association between the use of surgical sutures coated with an antimicrobial material to close the abdominal wound and surgical site infections. In a retrospective analysis, I compare a group receiving the coated sutures with a group that received the wound closure with a standard suture and I find a significant reduction in the wound infection rate in the patients that were treated with the coated suture. The two groups are well-balanced for several risk factors for wound infection such as age, sex, BMI, etc. *However, the proportion of patients with intra-operative contamination of the surgical field is significantly higher in the control group. Since contamination is an acknowledged risk factor for the outcome (wound infection), the association may be false. By stratifying the results for the confounder, it is possible to confirm or reject the association.*

By balancing the different prognosis factors across the groups, randomization partially prevents confounding bias. Randomization is not completely effective, however, because a certain amount of imbalance attributable to chance may occur. Confounding bias is a major risk in observational studies, especially owing to confounders that either are known but not considered or are unknown. Among all biases, confounding bias is the only one which can be partially corrected after completion of the study by statistical adjustment.

4.7.4 Other Types of Bias

In addition to the three types of bias described above, more specific biases exist that are related only to certain types of studies.

Diagnostic studies can have spectrum bias, a subtype of selection bias. The sensitivity and specificity of a diagnostic test can depend on who exactly is being tested. If only a section of the disease range is included in the study, for example, only the severe type, one may get a biased impression of how well a diagnostic test performs.

A final type of bias is not related to the study but to publication of the results. Numerous articles document the existence of "publication bias": studies with significant results are more easily published than those with negative (non-significant) findings. This bias, perhaps more appropriately called "negative-outcome bias," can occur at several levels: authors do not submit negative-outcome studies as often, reviewers do not recommend acceptance of negative-outcome studies as often, and editors may not accept negative-outcome studies as often. Even when published, negative studies are cited less frequently than positive studies. Publication and language biases can affect the results of literature reviews and meta-analyses.

There is a common misconception about biases: Retrospective studies are more biased than every other type of study, whereas randomized controlled trials do not experience bias owing to randomization. In retrospective studies, data on exposition and history often have been collected before the study was performed (i.e. in medical records) and therefore might be poorly standardized and more prone to classification bias. Nevertheless, a case–control study using well-standardized data or statistical methods to balance groups (i.e. propensity-matching analysis) should not experience more bias than a randomized study. Further, randomization does not totally prevent bias. Some biases do not depend on randomization, for example, attrition and classification biases which can be addressed by intent to treat analysis and blinding, respectively. Randomization only partially prevents selection and confounding biases; even if it usually produces comparable groups, a certain amount of covariate imbalance can still occur, especially when the sample size is small.

References

1. Wasserstein RL, Lazar NA. The ASA's statement on p-values: context, process, and purpose. Am Stat. 2016;70:129–33. https://doi.org/10.1080/00031305.2016.1154108.
2. Grabowsk B. "$P < 0.05$" might not mean what you think: American Statistical Association clarifies *P* values. J Natl Cancer Inst. 2016;108(8):djw194. https://doi.org/10.1093/jnci/djw194.
3. Wang M, Li D, Chen R, et al. Laparoscopic versus open pancreatoduodenectomy for pancreatic or periampullary tumours: a multicentre, open-label, randomised controlled trial. Lancet Gastroenterol Hepatol. 2021;6:438–47. https://doi.org/10.1016/S2468-1253(21)00054-6.
4. Sackett DL. Bias in analytic research. J Chronic Dis. 1979;32:51–63. https://doi.org/10.1016/0021-9681(79)90012-2.

Analyzing Continuous Variables: Descriptive Statistics, Dispersion and Comparison

5

Marco Ceresoli and Luca Nespoli

5.1 Introduction

A huge number of data, available every day in medical practice, can be collected and analyzed for various purposes such as observing the results of our practice, evaluating the impact of a technology, testing a new hypothesis. These data constitute only a limited sample from which we can try to obtain valid information about the entire population.

The aim of the chapter is to acquire some basic concepts regarding different types of data and variables we may encounter. The first important difference is between qualitative and quantitative variables.

We will discuss how to summarize and describe data and how to perform the appropriate analyses in order to reach the correct conclusions.

5.2 Qualitative Variables

Qualitative variables are non-numeric variables that describe an observation (not a measure) allocating it in several predetermined descriptive categories. Qualitative data are further divided into nominal and ordinal data. Ordinal data are divided into categories that could be ordered following some scale. The American Society of Anesthesiologists (ASA) score is an example of ordinal data: each patient could be classified into five fixed categories ordered from 1 to 5. It should be noticed that, despite represented by numeric values, ordinal variables are labels and should not be considered as numeric variables during statistical analysis. Another example is

M. Ceresoli (✉) · L. Nespoli
General and Emergency Surgery Department, School of Medicine and Surgery, Milano-Bicocca University, Monza, Italy
e-mail: marco.ceresoli@unimib.it

M. Ceresoli et al. (eds.), *Statistics and Research Methods for Acute Care and General Surgeons*, Hot Topics in Acute Care Surgery and Trauma,
https://doi.org/10.1007/978-3-031-13818-8_5

the tumor stage: patients can be allocated in four categories, that could be ordered, according to the tumor burden (stage I, stage II, stage III, stage IV).

Nominal data are data that can be allocated in categories, not necessarily numerical, that cannot be ordered, such as gender or surgical approach. These kind of variables (categorical) will be discussed in Chap. 6.

5.3 Quantitative Variables

Quantitative variables, also called numerical variables, are data measured and represented by a number. They are divided into discrete and continuous variables.

5.3.1 Discrete Variables

Discrete variables are data that could assume only a limited number of values and are represented by integers. An example is the injury severity score (ISS) in trauma patients, which could assume only an integer value between 0 and 75.

5.3.2 Continuous Variables

Continuous variables are data, derived from direct measurements, that can assume infinite values and may include decimals. Examples include weight and blood loss during surgery.

5.4 Describing Data

5.4.1 Data Distribution

A very important step in data description is the evaluation of their distribution. Data distribution represents the frequency on which each measure is recorded and it is considered when choosing the appropriate statistical test. There are two alternative scenarios: normally distributed data where data distribution follows predictable rules and non-normally distributed data, which are the most common in clinical practice.

Let us consider our hypothetical trauma register: we want to evaluate hemoglobin concentration in registered patients, a quantitative continuous variable.

The evaluation of data distribution could be easily done by a graphical representation through a histogram (see Fig. 5.1).

On the *X* axis the measures of Hb concentration are grouped in 0.5 g/dL intervals and ordered; on the *Y* axis is shown the frequency of observations for each group. In the example we can see that low and high values of Hb are observed less frequently and that the majority of observations are near "normal level" (between 12 g/dL and 16 g/dL). The distribution of observations is nearly symmetrical and the shape of

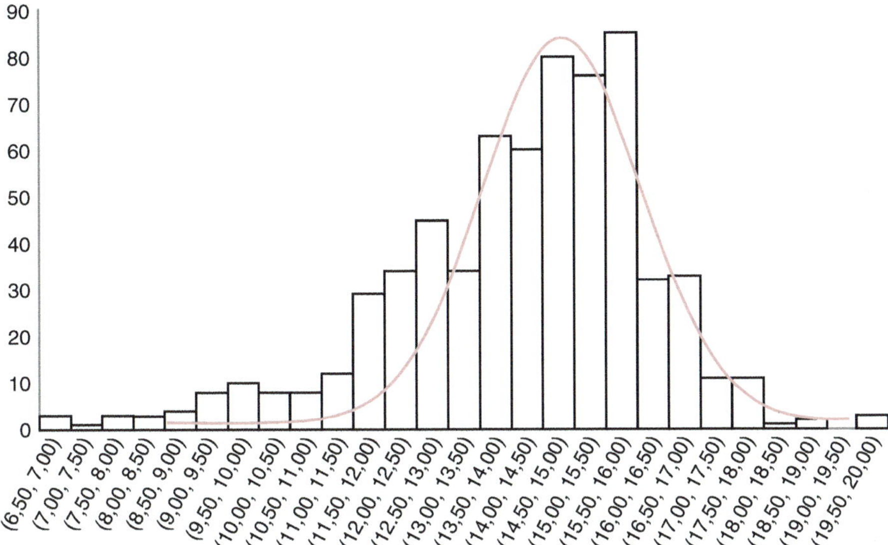

Fig. 5.1 Histogram of observed Hb concentration

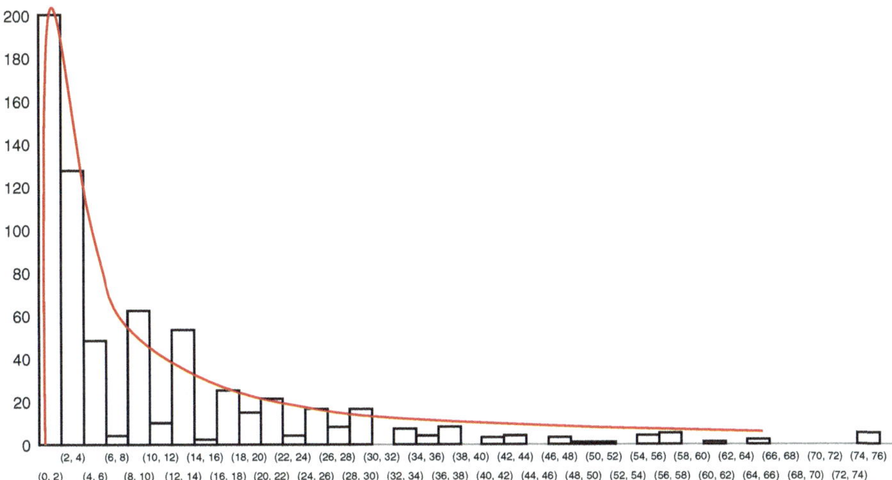

Fig. 5.2 Histogram of observed injury severity scores

the curve depicted by the histograms is "bell-shaped": this is a normal or Gaussian distribution.

We now want to assess the distribution of the injury Severity Score (ISS), a quantitative discrete variable, *collected* in our trauma register.

In this case (Fig. 5.2) the distribution of observations represented by the histograms is very different from a normal distribution as the majority of observations are located on the left side of the graph (low ISS). The shape of the curve traced along the histograms is not symmetric and there is a skewness, so that it is a non-normal distribution.

5.4.2 Test for Normality Assessment

The "normality" of data distribution, visually assessed with a histogram, can be evaluated through some statistic tests:

- The Shapiro–Wilk test is the most common test for normality assessment. It is based on the null hypothesis (H0) that our data have a normal distribution and it gives the probability that our data differ from the null hypothesis. With a low *p*-value ($p < 0.05$) we will reject the null hypothesis and conclude that our data do not follow a normal distribution. A $p > 0.05$ indicates normal distribution.
- The Kolmogorov–Smirnov normality test is a non-parametric test adopted for data comparison; it can be also adopted for evaluating the distribution of data. Similar to the Shapiro–Wilk test it tests the null hypothesis (H0: data normally distributed). With a *p*-value < of our alpha level (usually $p < 0.05$) we will reject the null hypothesis and we will conclude that our data are non-normally distributed. A $p > 0.05$ indicates normal distribution.

5.4.3 Descriptive Measures

The main purpose of descriptive statistics is to summarize all the observations into single measures. The most adopted descriptive measures are:

- Mean: This is the arithmetic mean and it is the value obtained from the sum of all the observed measures divided by the number of observations. It represents the average value of the observations and it is influenced by extremely large or small values of data. In Table 5.1 descriptive statistics of our example are reported. When data are normally distributed and are symmetrical such as hemoglobin concentration (Fig. 5.1), the mean is near equal to the median. In non-normally distributed data such as the ISS (Fig. 5.2) the mean value is 10.86 being influenced by some observations of large values. In this case the mean does not

Table 5.1 Example of descriptive and dispersion measures

		Normal distribution	Non-normal distribution
		Hemoglobin	ISS
Descriptive measures	Mean	14.25	10.86
	Median	14.60	5.00
Dispersion measures	Standard deviation	2.05	13.32
	25th percentile	13	2
	75th percentile	15.6	14

represent the "middle" value of data (the median ISS is 5) because the distribution of data and it is not symmetrical. The mean is the preferred and appropriate measure when data are normally distributed while it may be misleading when distribution of data is not symmetrical.

- Median: It corresponds to the "value in the middle" of our distribution of data, dividing the lower from the upper half of observations. In normally distributed data the median is equal to the mean. In our example the median ISS is 5: it means that 50% of the patients have an ISS equal or lower than the value 5. The mean in this case is very different (10.86) since it is influenced by the large values. In case of non-normally distributed data, the median is the preferred and appropriate measure to adopt.

5.4.4 Dispersion Measure

Mean and median are not sufficient to properly describe our data. For example, the two sets of data in Fig. 5.3 have the same mean but in one case data distribution is much narrower.

Therefore, for a complete description of our data we have to provide also a description of their dispersion, a measure that describes how much data differ from the mean. There are several measures to describe data dispersion. In this section we would briefly analyze the most commonly adopted:

- Variance: It is the arithmetic mean of the sum of the squares of the distance between each variable and the mean. It is not commonly adopted in scientific paper but is necessary to calculate the standard deviation and in other tests.
- Standard Deviation (also represented as SD or with the Greek letter σ): It is the commonest adopted measure of data dispersion and it is obtained by calculating the root square of the variance. It is expressed in the same unit of measure of the variable and it indicates how much data spread from the mean value. A high SD indicates a great dispersion with high variability, while a low SD represents a narrow distribution. It is the appropriate measure of data dispersion in case of normally distributed data. Since the distribution is normal and symmetrical we

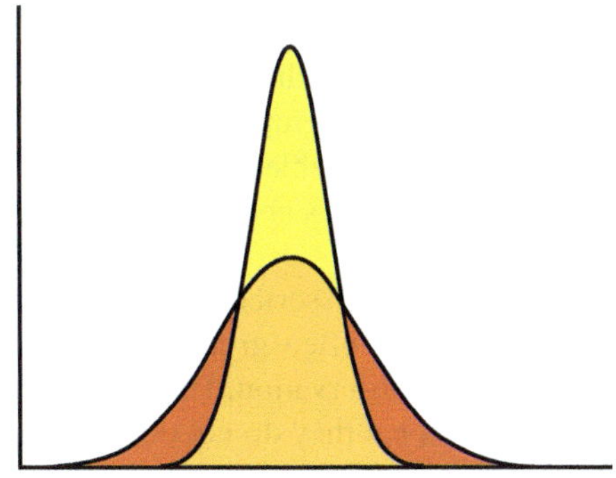

Fig. 5.3 An example of two sets of data with the same mean

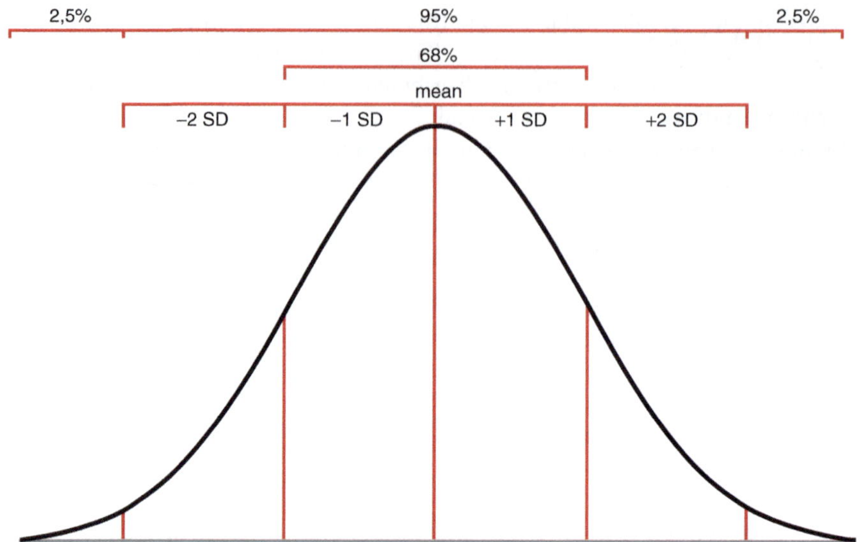

Fig. 5.4 A normal distribution, the mean and standard deviation (SD). 68% of the results are contained between the mean ± 1 SD; 95% of the results are contained between mean ± 2 SD

can indicate the mean followed by the standard deviation with the ± sign (mean ± SD). In normally distributed data 95% of the results are "contained" between ±2 SD (see Fig. 5.4).

- Interquartile Range (IQR): This is the preferred measure in case of non-normally distributed data and it is showed after the median (median (IQR)). It is obtained calculating the data distribution and percentiles, values below which a given percentage falls. The median is the 50th percentile (the value below which stays 50% of the observed values). The interquartile range is the range between the first quartile (25th percentile) and the third quartile (75th percentile). In our example (Table 5.1) the median ISS is 5 with an IQR (2–14).

5.4.5 Graphical Representations

Graphical representation is a very useful method to visualize and understand data and also to show results. Data distribution and descriptive statistics help in identifying the appropriate graph.

Continuous variables may also be resumed in tables with the abovementioned descriptive measures and dispersion measures. The most adopted graphs are:

- Histogram: It describes the distribution of data. On the *X* axis there are all the observations, often grouped, and for each one on the *Y* axis is shown the frequency of observation. Histograms provide useful information about data characteristics but they do not directly show descriptive and dispersion measure.

- Boxplot or Box and Whiskers Plot: It is the preferred graph to show continuous variables, especially if non-normally distributed. The height of the box, delimitated by the first and third quartiles (25th and 75th percentiles) represents the IQR. Inside the box is represented the median value. The two vertical lines beyond the box represent the minimum and maximum values contained within the limit of 1.5 IQR, while values outside this limit are defined as outliers and represented as dots. Figure 5.5 shows the boxplot of the injury severity score (ISS) in our trauma register (Table 5.1). Maximum and minimum in this graph do not correspond to the real maximum and minimum data but they are the maximum and minimum values contained within the limit of 1.5 IQR. All the other values are defined as "outlier" and are depicted as dots. In our example we can

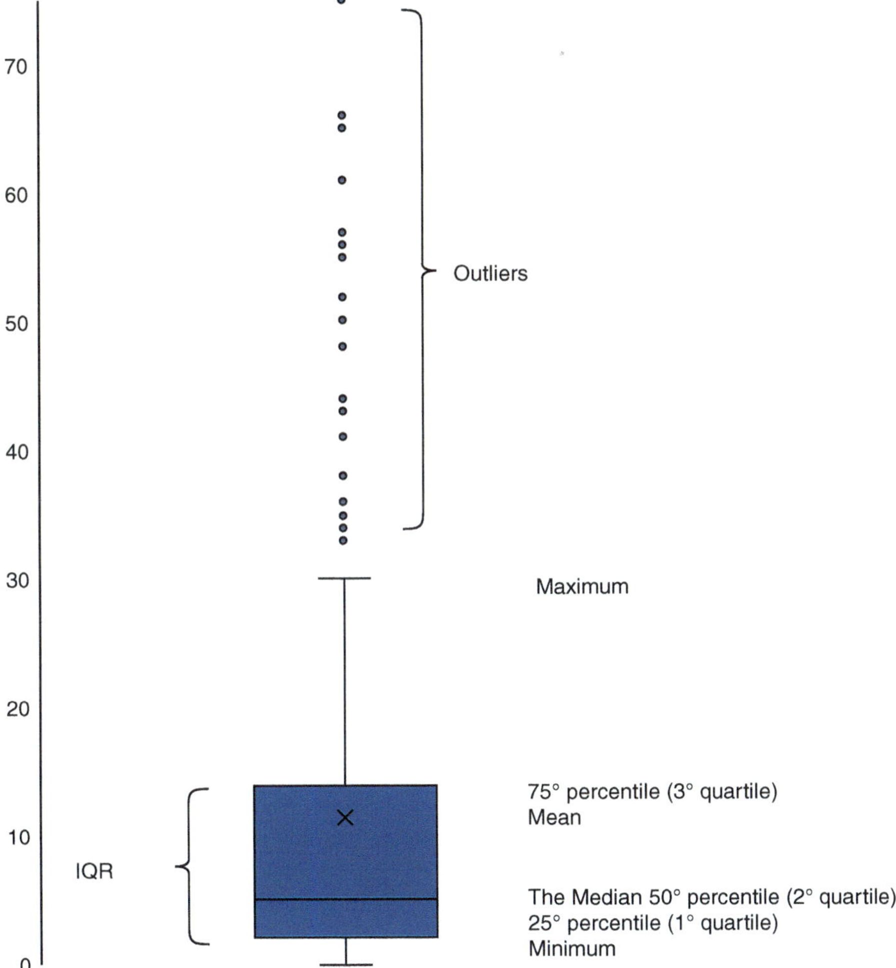

Fig. 5.5 Boxplot of the injury severity score

see how the data distribution is not symmetrical: the median value is not equidistant from the first and third quartiles.

5.5 Data Comparison: It Is All About Probability

In the previous section we have understood how continuous data may distribute and how they can be properly described. The majority of researches and studies have the aim to demonstrate the difference (superiority or inferiority) or the absence of difference (non-inferiority) between two or more samples of data such as patients' age or BMI, results of interventions, outcomes, etc. As explained in this chapter, it is all about probability. Statistical tests are based on hypothesis testing between the null (H0) hypothesis, which states that the two (or more) samples are equal, and the H1 hypothesis, which states that the samples are different. The concept is not immediate to understand and we have to make a "reductio ad absurdum (reduction to absurdity)": the test assumes that the H0 hypothesis is true and it gives us the probability to make an error in refusing the H0 hypothesis (concluding that samples are different each other) when it is correct (type 1 error – α). Usually an error up to 5% ($\alpha = 0.05$) is tolerated. A *p*-value of 0.01 represents a 1% probability of type 1 error; a *p*-value of 0.15 represents a 15% probability to refuse the H0 hypothesis when it is true.

From a practical point of view, when we observe two samples and we find a difference between them, the *p*-value gives us the probability that the observed difference is caused by a sampling imprecision and not because a true difference between the two samples exists. A low *p*-value means that this probability is very low and we can conclude (with a reasonable certainty) that the observed difference is true. A high *p*-value (generally >0.05, more than 5%) means that the probability that the observed difference is caused by a sampling problem is too high to conclude that it is true; therefore, we have to accept the null hypothesis and conclude that the two samples are similar.

For example: we want to compare the age between men and women admitted to our trauma center. We observed that mean age of men is 46.98 ± 19.08 years and women's mean age is 48.78 ± 18.45 years. The test gives us as result, a *p*-value of 0.354. The correct interpretation of this result is that the observed difference in terms of age has a 35.4% probability to be caused by a sampling problem and not by real difference among data. We cannot assume a real difference between the samples and we have to refuse the H1 hypothesis (ages are different) and to accept the null hypothesis.

5.5.1 Paired Data vs. Independent Data

Observed data can be classified into paired and independent data; this distinction is very important to choose the correct test to compare them.

We define paired data all the observations made in the same group of patients in two different time points (before and after an event), comparative statistics test the hypothesis of a difference between paired data. An example of paired data is the mean arterial pressure of trauma patients on the scene of trauma and at the arrival at the emergency department. Comparative statistics test the hypothesis of a difference between the sample of data before and after the treatment in the same group of patients.

Independent data are data collected from two or more different groups of patients, comparative statistics test the hypothesis of a difference between the groups. An example is the mean arterial pressure at the arrival at emergency department of patients with head trauma compared with patients without head trauma.

To compare the effect of a specific treatment before and after its application (paired data) in two different groups of patients (unpaired data) we have to adopt specific techniques such as "difference in difference" techniques that will be discussed in Chap. 13.

5.5.2 Parametric vs. Non-Parametric Statistics

Statistics tests are based on several assumptions. On the base of the assumptions needed we can describe two groups of tests: parametric and non-parametric tests.

Parametric tests imply the assumption that data have a normal distribution, they usually are more powerful and precise than non-parametric tests but they can be applied **only** if data follow a normal distribution (a relatively rare circumstance in clinical research).

Non-parametric tests are indicated when data do not follow a parameterized distribution (non-normal distribution): they do not need the assumption of normal distribution and they are generally widely usable but less powerful.

5.5.3 Commonest Tests

The following are the most common tests in clinical practice; they are based on hypothesis testing (H0 vs. H1) and provide a *p*-value as result to be interpreted. Table 5.2 contains the indications of the tests.

Table 5.2 Summary of statistics and their indications

Data distribution	Descriptive statistics	Data dispersion	Comparison test
Normal (parametric)	Mean	Standard deviation (±SD)	Student *t* test
Non-normal (non-parametric)	Median	Interquartile range (IQR)	Mann–Whitney *U* test

Table 5.3 Example of continuous variable comparison

Variable	Women	Men	p-value
Hemoglobin (normal distribution)	13.20 (±2.17) (mean ± SD)	14.50 (±2.12) (mean ± SD)	<0.001 (Student's t test)
ISS (non-normal distribution)	11.5 (5–19) (median (IQR))	12 (6–21) (median (IQR))	0.213 (Mann–Whitney U test)

- Student's t Test: This is the most known test for means comparison. Student's t test is a parametric test and it is appropriate when data follow a normal distribution. Student's t test applies on independent data (independent t test) and paired data (paired t test).
- Mann–Whitney's U Test: It compares two samples and it is indicated for non-parametric data.
- ANOVA: The term "anova" is the acronym of "ANalysis Of Variance." This is a very large and complex group of statistics based on the analysis of variance (a measure of data dispersion) that allows to make multiple comparisons (two or more groups, two or more hypothesis). This is an advanced statistics and we will not describe more deeply.

For example: We want to compare and evaluate if there is any difference between men and women admitted at our trauma center in age and injury severity score (ISS). Table 5.3 shows the characteristics of our population divided by patient sex.

In Table 5.3 the appropriate descriptive statistics for the two variables are shown. Hemoglobin concentration has a normal distribution (Fig. 5.1), therefore is represented with mean and standard deviation (SD). Data are compared with a parametric test, the Student's t test and the p-value show us that the difference observed is true with a probability >99% (1 − $p$value). Despite the statistical significance in the difference observed the interpretation of the test should take in count also the clinical significance: is a difference of 1.3 g/dL of Hb clinically significant?

The second line show data about the injury severity score, a non-normally distributed variable (see Fig. 5.2) that is described with the appropriate descriptive measure: the median along with interquartile range (IQR). In this case the non-parametric test for comparative data is the Mann–Whitney's U test that resulted in a p-value of 0.213. In this case the (slight) difference observed in ISS between men and women does not reach the statistical significance and we can conclude that in our trauma center men and women have similar ISS.

5.6 Linear Correlation

Continuous variables may be evaluated through linear correlation, the presence of linear relationship between two variables when data are graphically represented in a scatter graph where each variable is represented as a dot.

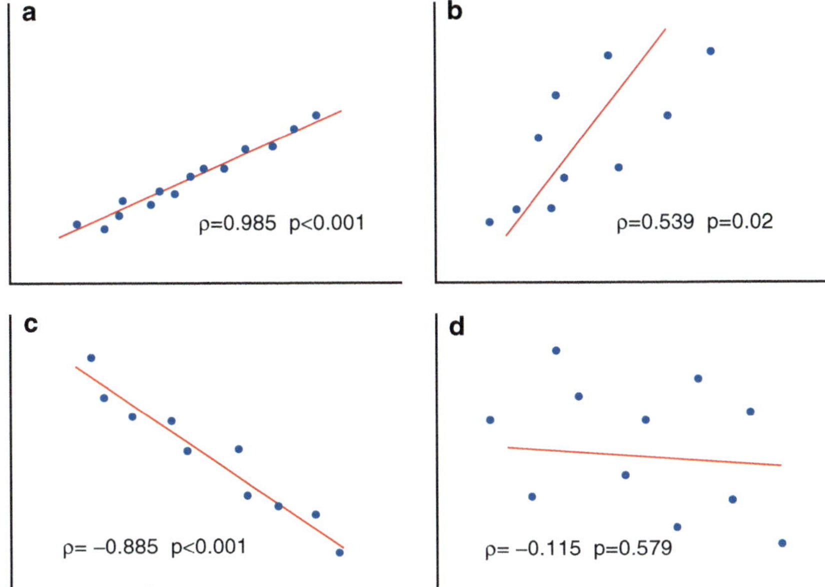

Fig. 5.6 (**a–d**)Four examples of linear correlations

5.6.1 Pearson Correlation

This relationship between two continuous variables is described by Pearson's correlation coefficient (or Pearson's ρ or correlation coefficient) that depends on the data dispersion (covariance and standard deviation). The Pearson's coefficient can assume a value between −1 and + 1. The value +1 corresponds to a positive perfectly linear relation, the value −1 to a negative perfectly linear relation, and a value 0 means no linear relation. Figure 5.6 shows different scenarios of linear correlation.

In example "a" data have a near perfectly positive linear relation and the ρ coefficient is approximatively 1. In example "C" there is a similar linear relationship but negative and ρ is negative. In example "b" the linear relation is less perfect than example "A" and the ρ coefficient is 0.539. In example "d" it is evident that there is no linear relation between data and the ρ coefficient is near zero.

5.6.2 Pearson Coefficient Interpretation

As stated before, the Pearson's correlation coefficient can assume values between +1 and −1. As a rule of thumb the correlation coefficient can be interpreted as follows:

Positive correlation	Negative correlations	Strength
0.7–1	−0.7 to −1	Strong correlation
0.3–0.7	−0.3 to −0.7	Moderate correlation
0.1–0.3	−0.3 to 0.1	Weak correlation

The coefficient is followed by the significance level (*p*-value) that indicates the certainty or uncertainty of the relationship observed.

It is to notice that the correlation coefficient does not indicate the slope of the linear relation: in example "a" the coefficient is near 1 that indicates a near perfect linear relationship. Looking to the slope of the identified linear relation, in example "b" the slope is higher than in example "a," but the correlation coefficient is lower. Pearson's correlation is influenced by the data dispersion and not by the slope of the correlation (it will be evaluated with linear regression, Chap. 9).

5.6.3 Spearman's Rank Correlation Coefficient

Spearman's rank correlation is the statistical method used to evaluate the linear correlation between two discrete or continuous ordinal set of data. Its interpretation is very similar to the interpretation of Pearson's linear correlation.

Further Reading

Altman DG. Practical statistics for medical research. London: Chapman & Hall; 1991.
Kirkwood BR, Sterne JAC. Essential medical statistics. Oxford: Blackwell; 2003.
Walters SJ, Campbell MJ, Machin D. Medical statistics. Chichester: Blackwell; 2021.

6 Analyzing Categorical Variable: Descriptive Statistics and Comparisons

Alessandro Cucchetti

6.1 Introduction

In general, categorical data provides information on frequency, information on the proportion, or the presence or absence of a particular result in an observation. Before explaining the descriptive and comparative approaches for categorical variables, it is necessary to explain three terms: categorical variable, categories, and categorical data [1]. Suppose there are both boys and girls in a class. In this case, gender is a **categorical variable** with two **categories** under the gender variable, namely male and female. The frequencies associated with each category are **categorical data**. According to Stevens' theory of measurement (1946), categorical variables are measured at the nominal level. The nominal level is a measurement scale in which numbers serve as labels to classify an object. However, also variables measured at the ordinal level can be considered categorical variables. For example, in a classroom about 3% of students receive an A, 15% a B, 64% a C, 15% a D, and the remaining 3% an E (Table 6.1). The rating scale conveys an **ordinal** type of information but it can also be treated as a **categorical variable** of nominal level for which the frequency of students who receive one of these five grades is tabulated and analyzed.

To deal with nominal and ordinal data, it is useful to tabulate frequencies of occurrences in each category while simultaneously converting frequencies into proportions. A **one-way table** refers to a display of frequencies based on a single

A. Cucchetti (✉)
Department of Medical and Surgical Sciences—DIMEC,
Alma Mater Studiorum—University of Bologna, Bologna, Italy

Morgagni—Pierantoni Hospital, Forlì, Italy
e-mail: alessandro.cucchett2@unibo.it

M. Ceresoli et al. (eds.), *Statistics and Research Methods for Acute Care and General Surgeons*, Hot Topics in Acute Care Surgery and Trauma,
https://doi.org/10.1007/978-3-031-13818-8_6

Table 6.1 The rating scale conveys an ordinal type of information ranging from A to E but it can also be treated as a categorical variable, thus observed proportions are calculated

Rate	Number of cases	Observed proportions (%)	Expected proportions (%)	(Expected – observed)^2/expected
A	3	3	20	289/20
B	15	15	20	25/20
C	64	64	20	1936/20
D	15	15	20	25/20
E	3	3	20	289/20
Total	100	100	100	128.2

Under the assumption that proportions would be equal, each rate would contain 20 cases. The chi-squared test for goodness of fit relies on the comparison between observed and expected proportions. The degrees of freedom are the number of categories minus 1 (df = 4). Having known the χ^2 and the df, *p*-value can be derived from conversion tables [2]

categorical variable. A **two-way table** is a tabulation of joint frequencies of two variables. Usually, a two-way table uses one dimension, such as columns, to represent one variable and another dimension, such as rows, to represent the second variable. Similarly, a **multi-way** table involves three or more categorical variables and its commonly presented on the output as several two-way tables segregated by the third variable (or vice versa).

A one-way table displays categorical data in the form of frequency counts and/or relative frequencies. It has a descriptive purpose only but statistical analysis can be performed through the comparison of the **observed** versus **expected** proportions. Considering that the classroom receiving rates are formed by 100 students, it would be useful in some instances to verify if observed versus expected proportions fulfill the equal distribution of proportions. If this latter condition is theoretically present, each category (five categories) should have 100/5 = 20 cases each. However, we know that this is not true, and the chi-square test provides a measure of such a different distribution. In this specific case, the chi-square test of equal proportions (namely chi-squared test for goodness of fit) is statistically significant ($\chi^2 = 128.2$, degree of freedom [df] = 4, $p < 0.001$). Therefore, the null hypothesis of equal proportions of students in each of the rating categories is rejected at $\alpha = 0.05$.

6.2 Confidence Interval of Proportions

Another important descriptive data for categories is the calculation of **confidence intervals** (CI) for proportions. This informs you the statistical probability that a characteristic is likely to occur within the population. For example, consider that the percentage of students receiving a C is 64% (p = 0.640) among 100 students (n = 100). The CI for this proportion is calculated with two bounds: the lower bound is 0.546 and the upper bound is 0.734.

This means that if the rating of students is repeated over and over again, the results would fall within 54.6% and 73.4% 95% of the time. Larger the sample size, narrow the confidence range.

6.3 Absolute Risk Reduction and Number Needed-to-Treat

When dealing with a **two-way** table, other considerations should be made. Suppose that your study, comparing treatment A versus treatment B, finally shows that 20% treated with A developed bad outcomes, whereas only 10% of those receiving treatment B developed bad outcomes. It appears that treatment B can reduce some of the bad outcomes of the disease and this difference can be quantified using different measures [3]. The **absolute risk reduction** (ARR) is also called risk difference (RD) and it is simply calculated as the difference among two proportions, that is, the ARR of B over A is 20% − 10% = 10%. This means that, if 100 patients were treated, 10 would be prevented from experiencing bad outcomes if treatment B is adopted. Another way of expressing this is the **number needed-to-treat** (NNT). This is simply = 1/ARR so that in this hypothetical scenario NNT = 1/0.10 = 10, that is, every 10 patients treated with treatment B, one additional would benefit from B rather than A. Conventionally, an NNT <5 rules in therapies with high gains, whereas an NNT > 15 rules out therapies with low health gain [4].

6.4 Relative Risk and Relative Risk Reduction

Some other measures are commonly used. The **relative risk** (RR) of a bad outcome in a group given treatment A is a proportional measure which estimates the size of the effect of treatment A compared with treatment B. It is the proportion of bad outcomes in the intervention group divided by the proportion of bad outcomes in the control group. In the above hypothetical case, the RR is 0.5 (10%/20% = 0.5). When a treatment has an RR > 1, the risk of a bad outcome is increased by the treatment; when RR < 1, the risk of a bad outcome is decreased, meaning that the treatment is likely to do good. For example, when the RR is 2.0 the chance of a bad outcome is twice as likely to occur with a specific treatment as without it. In the present hypothetical scenario, the RR was 0.5 meaning that the chance of a bad outcome is halved with treatment B compared to treatment A. A value of RR = 1.2 means that exposed people are 20% more likely to have bad outcome, RR = 1.4 means 40% more likely. When the RR is exactly 1, the risk is unchanged.

Relative risk reduction (RRR) informs about how much the treatment reduced the risk of bad outcomes relative to the control group who did not have that specific treatment. In the previous example, the RRR of bad outcomes can be calculated as (20% − 10%)/10% = 100%. This means that treatment B decreases bad outcomes with a magnitude of 100% with respect to treatment B.

6.5 Odds Ratio

Odds of a specific outcome is the ratio between the probability of the outcome and the probability of not occurring in this outcome [5]. Thus, differently from RR, **odds ratio** (OR) considers the number of subjects without the specific outcome of interest. Rare diseases yield similar risk and odds since the number of non-cases is close to the number of subjects but for common diseases, risk and odds can differ considerably. Consider that treatment A produced a bad outcome in 20% out of 100 patients, and that treatment B produced a bad outcome in 10% out of 100 patients, this means that:

a = number of exposed to treatment A cases = 20.
b = number of exposed to treatment A non-cases = 80.
c = number of non-exposed to treatment A cases = 10.
d = number of non-exposed to treatment A cases = 90.

Odds ratio derives from $(a/c)/(b/d)$, that is, the ratio between cases and non-cases of exposed and non-exposed. In the present hypothetical example, OR can be calculated as follows:

$$(20/10)/(80/90) = 2/0.889 = 2.25.$$

As can be noted OR is different from the previous RR = 2.0 because it answers to a different question. Relative risk gives you the ratio among proportions, whereas OR gives you the ratio of a probability but the interpretation is similar, that is, the probability (odds) of bad outcome is 2.25 times higher among patients exposed to treatment A compared to treatment B. Odds ratio is more informative than RR because it considers the sample size of the population.

6.6 Chi-Squared Test and Fisher's Exact Test

When we try to compare proportions of a categorical outcome according to different independent groups, we can consider several statistical tests such as chi-squared test and Fisher's exact test [6]. The chi-squared test and Fisher's exact test can assess the independence between two variables when the comparing groups are not correlated, thus independent of each other. The chi-squared test applies an approximation assuming the sample is large, while the Fisher's exact test runs an exact procedure. The difference is simply related to the elaboration required to compute the Fisher's exact test. When modern calculators were still not available, Fisher's exact test was time-consuming, so that a good approximation was obtained through Pearson's chi-squared test. To date, Fisher's exact test should be preferred over chi-squared, especially when more than 20% of cells of a 2 × 2 contingency table have expected frequencies <5, because applying approximation method is inadequate.

Requirements for computing **chi-squared test** are: that the sample is picked at random, that observations must be independent of each other (so, for example, no matched pairs), and that cell count must be 5 or above for each cell in a 2 × 2 contingency table. For the previous hypothetical case of treatment A versus treatment B, all cells (a, b, c, d) contain >5 cases, and data are not matched so that chi-squared can be applied. The chi-square statistic is = 3.9216 with a p-value = 0.047. To reduce the error in approximation, Frank Yates suggested a correction named **Yates correction** that adjusts the Pearson's chi-squared test formula by subtracting 0.5 from the difference between each observed value and its expected value in a 2 × 2 contingency table. In the previous case, the chi-square statistic with Yates correction is 3.176 and the p-value is 0.074. Applying the Fisher's exact test, the p-value is 0.073. It becomes clear that Fisher's exact test and Yates correction of the chi-squared are more conservative approaches to verify a hypothesis about difference, but Fisher's has to be preferred because it is an exact test and not an approximation.

6.7 Matched Data

The chi-squared test and Fisher's exact test require that observations must be independent of each other. If data are not dependent, another approach must be adopted. The **McNemar** test is used to determine if there are differences in a dichotomous dependent variable between two related groups. It can be considered to be similar to the paired-samples t-test, but for a dichotomous rather than a continuous dependent variable. The McNemar test is particularly useful when dealing with propensity score match, since due to the matched nature of propensity score approach, this should be considered as the most appropriate statistical analysis to adopt.

6.8 Chi-Squared Test for Trend

When dealing with more than two groups, one can have interest in verifying if a specific outcome has an association with the different groups considered, ranked in a pre-specified order. In the example of student rating, there was not any trend in proportion moving from A to E. Suppose now to have four groups (Table 6.2). The first is formed by patients treated with treatment A between 2006 and 2009, the second is formed by those treated between 2010 and 2013, the third is formed by

Table 6.2 Odds ratio values are calculated for each stratum against the first period (2006–2009)

Period	Number of patients	Observed events/n	Frequency (%)	Observed non-events	Odds ratio
2006–2009	25	8	32	17	1
2010–2013	25	6	24	19	0.67
2014–2017	25	4	16	21	0.40
2018–2021	25	2	8	23	0.18
Total	100	20	20	80	–

The Mantel–Haenszel test of trend highlights if there is a linear association among OR variations. As can be noted, in comparison to the first period, ORs progressively decreased with the passing of time, and this is the trend detected by the test those treated between 2014 and 2017, and the last is formed by those treated between 2018 and 2021. Bad outcomes occurred in 20% among 100 patients between 2006 and 2021, but the proportion was 32% in the first period (i.e. 8/25), decreased to 24% in the second period (i.e. 6/25), then further decreased to 16% (i.e. 4/25) in the third period and was finally 8% in the most recent period (i.e. 2/25). The simple application of a chi-squared test will verify if that proportions are equal or not among different period considered. For this specific example, the chi-square statistic is 5 with a *p*-value = 0.172. This did not consider the trend over time. This is accomplished by the **Mantel–Haenszel test of trend** among chi-squared test statistics [7]. This test returns a chi-square statistic extended for trend of 5.46 with a *p*-value = 0.019.

6.9 Standardized Differences

This measure overcomes problems related to the sample of the population analyzed [8]. Considering bad outcomes of treatment A versus treatment B, that is, 20% versus 10%. The **ARR** is 10%. Until now we considered 100 patients per group so that applying the Fisher's exact test, the *p*-value was 0.073. Suppose to increase the sample to 1000 patients per group, maintaining fixed 20% and 10% of bad outcomes. Under this last circumstance, Fisher's exact test returns a *p*-value <0.001. Thus, the larger the sample, the lower the *p*-value but the **ARR** remains as 10%, as well as **RR** and **OR**. The question is not if treatment A is superior to treatment B, but what is the magnitude of this difference. This can be assessed by standardized difference, commonly abbreviated as **d-value**, a dimensionless measure that is independent from the sample size.

The standardized difference was proposed in the psychological literature, where it has been referred to as Cohen's Effect Size Index [9]. Cohen suggested that Effect Size Indices of 0.2, 0.5, and 0.8 can be used to represent small, medium, and large effect sizes, respectively [9]. When the two populations being considered are normally distributed with equal variance and are of the same size, Cohen derived relationships between the *d*-value and the percentage of overlap cases and the probability of superiority of one treatment over the alternative [10]. In the present hypothetical case the % of overlap was 88.9% and the probability of superiority was 57.8%. A treatment without any effect will have a % of overlap of 100% and a probability of superiority of 50% (the toss of a coin).

References

1. Peng CY. Categorical data analysis. In: Data analysis using SAS®. Thousand Oaks, CA: SAGE; 2009. p. 239–90. https://doi.org/10.4135/9781452230146.
2. Social Science Statistics. https://www.socscistatistics.com/pvalues/chidistribution.aspx. Accessed 23 Oct 2021.

3. Ranganathan P, Pramesh CS, Aggarwal R. Common pitfalls in statistical analysis: absolute risk reduction, relative risk reduction, and number needed to treat. Perspect Clin Res. 2016;7:51–3. https://doi.org/10.4103/2229-3485.173773.
4. Chong CA, Tomlinson G, Chodirker L, Figdor N, Uster M, Naglie G, Krahn MD. An unadjusted NNT was a moderately good predictor of health benefit. J Clin Epidemiol. 2006;59:224–33. https://doi.org/10.1016/j.jclinepi.2005.08.005.
5. Szumilas M. Explaining odds ratios [published correction appears in J Can Acad Child Adolesc Psychiatry]. J Can Acad Child Adolesc Psychiatry. 2010;19:227–9.
6. Kim HY. Statistical notes for clinical researchers: Chi-squared test and Fisher's exact test. Restor Dent Endod. 2017;42:152–5. https://doi.org/10.5395/rde.2017.42.2.152.
7. Schlesselman S. Case-control studies. New York, Oxford: Oxford University Press; 1982. p. 203–6.
8. Austin PC. Balance diagnostics for comparing the distribution of baseline covariates between treatment groups in propensity-score matched samples. Stat Med. 2009;28:3083–107. https://doi.org/10.1002/sim.3697.
9. Cohen J. Statistical power analysis for the behavioral sciences. 2nd ed. Hillsdale: Lawrence Erlbaum; 1988.
10. Interpreting Cohen's d Effect Size. https://rpsychologist.com/cohend/. Accessed 23 Oct 2021.

Part III

Advanced Statistics

Multivariate Analysis

7

Niccolò Allievi and Marco Ceresoli

7.1 Introduction

7.1.1 Statistical Models

Describing reality essentially means building statistical models of observed biological events and processes. For clinicians, the prediction of outcomes depends on our capacity of establishing accurate models on observed data and therefore inferring information regarding the general population (the real world). The fit of our model to the observed data represents the accuracy to which the model represents the collected data and is of paramount importance for the overall validity of the description.

As surgeons, one of our aims is understanding the relationships between the characteristics of our patients and their outcomes. In order to do so, we build models describing a small proportion (i.e. the patients included in a trauma register) and we imply that our model also fits the "general population" (i.e. all patients who sustain a traumatic injury). The smaller the error intrinsic to the model, the higher the fit of the model: this is a key concept when building and evaluating statistical models.

Predicting outcomes with statistical models will contemplate three main steps:

- Building the model.
- Assessing the fit of the model.
- Interpreting the model.

N. Allievi (✉)
Surgical Department, Papa Giovanni XXIII Hospital, Bergamo, Italy

M. Ceresoli
General and Emergency Surgery Department, School of Medicine and Surgery, Milano-Bicocca University, Monza, Italy

M. Ceresoli et al. (eds.), *Statistics and Research Methods for Acute Care and General Surgeons*, Hot Topics in Acute Care Surgery and Trauma,
https://doi.org/10.1007/978-3-031-13818-8_7

7.1.2 Different Types of Regressions and Multiple Regression

Running a regression essentially means building a model to assess how one of the variables (the "outcome" variable) is associated with the other available variables (the "predictor" variables). Depending on the outcome variable, we need to choose among different types of regression:

- If the outcome variable is continuous, we will choose linear regression;
- If the outcome variable is binary, we will choose binary logistic regression;
- For categorical variables multinomial logistic regression would be the correct choice, but the statistical concepts are the same as for binary logistic regression.
- For other type of outcome variables exists specific regression models, for example, the ordinal regression for ordinal outcomes or the Poisson regression for frequency outcomes. These models are advanced and not frequent in surgical studies and will not be discussed in this chapter.

Depending on the number of predictors, we will have different kinds of regression. If there is one predictor in the model, this would be a "univariate" regression, while if more than one predictor is included in the model, we would build a "multivariable" or "multiple" regression.

Different (and somehow confusing) terms are used:

- Univariate regression: one outcome variable, one predictor;
- Multivariable (or multiple) regression: one outcome variable, several predictors;
- Multivariate (or multinomial) regression: several outcome variables (that will not be discussed in this chapter).

7.1.3 Example: The Dataset

To help clarify the concepts exposed in the chapter, we will refer to a practical example. Table 7.1 contains observed data of an imaginary database of patients who sustained traumatic injuries.

If we were to predict the length of stay as our outcome variable, notwithstanding the characteristics of the predictors, we would use a linear regression; on the

Table 7.1 Example dataset

ID	Age	Sex	ISS	Length of stay	Shock	ICU admission
1	80	Male	48	65	1	1
2	60	Male	29	30	1	1
3	55	Female	41	50	0	1
4	16	Male	5	4	0	0
5	20	Female	9	5	0	0
6	78	Female	14	10	1	1
...	...	...	...	...	...	...

contrary, if we wanted to predict ICU admission (0 = no admission versus 1 = admission), we would use a logistic regression model.

7.2 Linear Regression Models

7.2.1 Building a Linear Regression Model: It All Comes Down to the Straight Line Equation

Considering our example dataset, we can create a scatterplot of our observations, where the ISS is on the *X*-axis and the length of stay on the *Y*-axis. Our outcome is the length of stay, which is a continuous variable, and we want to study its relationship to another continuous variable, the burden of injury (the Injury Severity Score, namely ISS).

We can see there is a linear relationship between the predictor variable and the outcome variable, as the distribution of each value on the graph depicts a line. This line is the regression line.

All statistical models built to predict an outcome (*Yi*) are made of variables (*Xi*) and parameters (*bi*). Variables represent measurable elements in our population, while parameters are estimated from the data itself and describe the relationships between variables within the model. From a mathematical point of view our model will be similar to the equation of the straight line (line = intercept + slope × predictor). This in fact justifies the name "linear models." The intercept (*b*0) and the slope (*b*1) are the regression coefficients and they estimate the relationship between each of the parameters and the outcome:

- The intercept or constant (*b*0) represents the value of *Yi* where the line crosses the *Y*-axis; in other words, it is the value of the outcome when the predictor is equal to 0.
- The slope (gradient) of the line (*b*1) is the parameter estimate of the predictor and shows a positive or negative relationship between *Xi* and *Yi*.

When multiple predictors are used, multiple regression takes place: Each predictor variable (*Xi*) has a parameter (*b*) or regression coefficients. The parameters will describe the shape of the model in a geometrical space. When one predictor is used, we could represent our data as a scatterplot on a Cartesian 2D space; the result of a simple linear regression would be a straight line (a "fit line"). When two predictors are used (multiple linear regression), the data might be outlined in a 3D scatterplot and the model would fit with a "regression plane." If we add more predictors, it would be more difficult to represent the model geometrically.

7.2.2 Interpreting the Linear Regression Model

The interpretation of the model should be systematic. Let us see our example in Fig. 7.1.

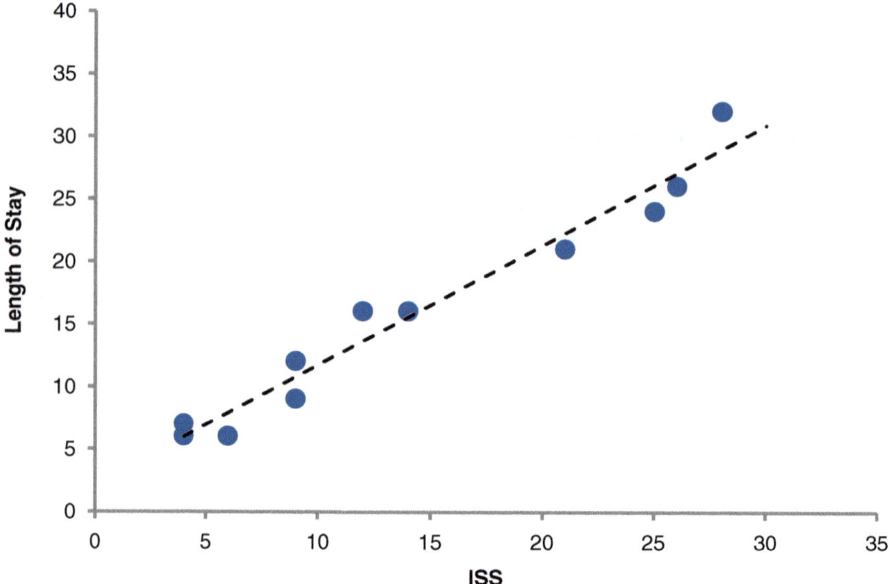

Fig. 7.1 A scatterplot showing the relationship between ISS and length of stay in the example

7.2.2.1 Interpreting the Parameters of the Model

- *b*0 is often reported as Beta0 (*β*0) and represents the value of the outcome variable when all variables are equal to zero (*Xi* = 0). Although this is often omitted, with *b*(0) it is possible to estimate the outcome variable giving the explanatory variables a specific value. In our example Beta0 is 1, which means that the predicted length of stay when the ISS is 0 is 1 day.
- *b* or Beta are usually reported for each predictor. Each *b* value gives an idea of the direction (positive or negative) and strength of the relationship between the predictor (*Xi*) and the outcome variable (*Yi*). Beta or *b* is a number and it could assume every value from $-\infty$ to $+\infty$. A value equal to zero represents no effect. A positive value (beta > 0) means a positive relationship between the dependent variable and the predictor with an increment equal to beta for each increment in the value of the predictor. A beta below 0 (beta < 0) represents a negative relationship between the dependent variable and the predictor, with a decrease equal to beta for each increment in the value of the predictor. The higher the value of beta, the greater the effect.
  - Continuous variable predictor: The beta number tells us that for every single increase in the predictor variable *Xi*, there is an increase equal to beta in the outcome variable. In our example *b*(ISS) = 1.22 (95% CI 1.05–1.40, *p*-value 0.001): for every increase of 1 in the ISS, the length of stay has an increment of 1.2 days; *b*(ISS) also represents the slope of the line in Fig. 7.1.
  - Categorical variable predictor: In case that predictor is a categorical variable, *b* indicates that cases expressing the predictor have, on average, *b* units of the

outcome variable in excess (or defect, depending on the sign of b), as compared to cases not expressing the predictor. In a hypothetical example b(men) = 1.9 (95% CI 1.45–2.37, p-value 0.001) means that men have a length of stay 1.9 longer compared to women.

7.2.2.2 Interpreting 95% Confidence Intervals

- Each parameter is reported along with the 95% confidence intervals that will estimate the interval for that single parameter of the slope; if the 95% CI crosses the value 0, this would impair statistical and clinical significance. An associated p value will give the degree of statistical significance. The degree of clinical significance will also be judged on the magnitude of the effect. The 95% CI for b(ISS) and b(men) does not cross 0 and the p-values are <0.05; we can state that the associations between ISS and sex with the length of stay are statistically significant.

Furthermore, it should be reminded that the interpretation of data should be kept within the range of values of the independent variable (ISS). It is not directly possible to extrapolate values of the dependent variable, when outside the "sown field" of observed explanatory variables (for instance, in our dataset our maximum ISS was 48 and we cannot comment on patients with a higher ISS).

Finally, regression coefficients are "just" slopes: their magnitude depends on the unit used to measure the outcome variable and the predictor variable(s). We can appreciate this if we change the measure unit for our length of stay to hours or minutes: the results of the slopes would be macroscopic.

7.2.3 Assumptions of Linear Regression

We now outline the main assumptions of linear regression. Without these assumptions being fulfilled a linear regression would be not appropriate. All of these aspects are advanced statistics and will not be described exhaustively.

- *Linearity*: The predicted variable (Yi) should be linearly related to the predictor(s) (Xi). This can be verified visually on a scatterplot of observed data. If linearity is violated, the variables might be transformed (e.g. logarithmic transformation) before proceeding with the analysis.
- *Normally distributed errors*: Residuals in the model are normally distributed.
- *Independent observations*: Each case needs to have a single observation for the dependent variable and a single observation for the independent variable for each analysis that is performed.
- *Homoscedasticity*: Residuals at every level of the dependent variable(s) should have the same variance, i.e. the variance of the residuals is the same for every value of X. Looking at the scatterplot will give a glimpse regarding the constancy of variation within observed Y values throughout the "X spectrum." When this is violated, possible solutions are: transformation of the outcome variable; stratification of data on the predictor variable or on the outcome variable.

7.3 Multiple Regression

Simple linear regression evaluates the relation between a single predictor and the outcome. It could be repeated for each predictor, giving results of "*univariate*" analysis. In fact these (univariate) analyses do not take count of the possible relations between predictors.

Multiple regressions are indicated to evaluate also the possible relations among predictors and give a stronger evidence, adjusted for possible confounders.

Multiple regression models require a careful and accurate choice of predictors to be inserted in the model. This is a crucial step since the results will depend on the predictors.

7.3.1 Choice of Predictors

When running a multiple regression, the choice of the dependent variables (X) is extremely important. Regarding the numerosity of the variables, as a rule of thumb we need at least 10 outcomes events or cases for every predictor variable and 10 for the intercept, although the sample size depends mainly on the effect size we are trying to detect and on the statistical power. If too many predictors are fitted into the model, the result would be overfitting of the model: one of the possible complications is that the model is going to detect idiosyncrasies, which are not truly present in the observed data.

As another rule of thumb, it is quite accepted among researchers to include in the multiple regression model all the predictors resulted associated with the outcome at the univariate phase of the analysis: all the variables with p-values <0.05 at univariate analysis should be included; furthermore, the variables that resulted to have a satisfactory clinical significance at univariate analysis, also with a borderline statistical significance (e.g. p-values around 0.1), should be considered for inclusion in the multiple regression. In general, it is believed that parsimony is key when choosing predictors. If a biological event can be explained by several models, the simpler one would probably be preferable. While developing multivariable models, we should select explanatory variables by the degree of contribution they give to explain reality. It is also worth mentioning that, whenever an interaction between two explanatory variables is reported, this interaction should be included in the model, whatever the level of contribution.

Several approaches to variable selection are described:

- *Stepwise approach*:
  - Forward method: To an initial model only containing $b0$ (the constant), predictors are added one by one and the model fit is evaluated repeatedly, until a good model is found. Some software may run an automated forward linear regression: the criterion used to select the variables to include is to maximize R^2 (a measure of the fit of the model). This method might be flawed by the absence of clinical significance and by potentially detrimental correlation between the variables.

– Backward method: an initial model containing as many predictors as possible is created and the model fit is maximized removing single predictors in several steps.

- *Hierarchical approach*: The initial model includes significant predictors that were previously included in research studies with sound methodology or that carry known clinical relevance (a priori decision regarding the essential selection of variables). Single predictors may be added to this model and model fit can be re-evaluated serially. This is, in general, the preferred approach by many researchers.
- *Forced entry approach*: The predictor variables are added all in one model and its validity is tested.

Finally, apart from the variable of interest of the study, established confounders for the outcome of interest should always be included in the study.

7.3.1.1 Example: Inclusion of Predictors for Multivariable Analysis

We are now interested in exploring the association between our outcome variable (length of stay) and other possible predictors in the dataset, such as the ISS, age, sex, and shock condition. We therefore run linear univariate analysis for each predictor and the results are as follows (Table 7.2): *b*(ISS) = 1.22 (95% CI 1.05–1.40, *p*-value 0.001); *b*(age) = −0.8 (95% CI −1.2 to 0.4, *p*-value 0.002); *b*(man) = 1.9 (95% CI 1.45–2.37, *p*-value 0.001), and *b*(shock) = 1.16 (95% CI −1.5 to 2.6 *p*-value 0.087). The regression coefficients for age, sex, and ISS are clinically and statistically significant, while we can see that the 95% CI for shock condition crosses 0 and that the associated *p*-value is >0.05. We will therefore include only age, sex, and ISS in the multivariable analysis.

Table 7.2 shows the results of the univariate analysis (for each predictor, left side of the table) and the results of the multivariable linear regression in the right side of the table. We can notice that beta coefficients, 95% confidence intervals, and *p*-value are shown only for predictors included in the multiple analysis. The multiple linear regression shows us that only ISS and sex are related with the length of stay.

Table 7.2 Essential elements to report results of a univariate and a multivariable linear regression, using results from the example dataset

Independent variables	Dependent variable (length of stay)—univariate regression			Dependent variable (length of stay)—multiple regression		
	b (or Beta)	95% CI	*p*-value	*b* (or Beta)	95% CI	*p*-value
Constant (*b*0)	0.98	–	–	1.07	–	–
ISS	1.22	1.05–1.40	0.001	1.21	0.80–1.41	0.001
Age	−0.8	−1.2 to 0.4	0.002	−0.6	−1.2 to 1.12	0.465
Sex (men)	1.9	1.45–2.37	0.001	1.4	1.2–1.8	0.02
Shock	1.16	−1.5 to 2.6	0.087	–		

If we consider the ISS as the main predictor being investigated in the study, we can state that the correlation between the ISS and the length of stay remained true also after correction for confounders, i.e. the age and the sex. For each increment in the ISS we would observe an increment of 1.21 days in the length of stay; men would experience a longer length of stay of 1.4 days when compared with women.

7.3.2 Adjustment for Confounders

Another way of looking at multivariable analysis is the following: the aim of multiple regression is to determine an independent relationship of a variable of interest with an outcome, by accounting for other factors that may influence the association, which are known as "confounders." A confounder is a variable that is associated with the main variable of interest (the main risk factor), without being affected by the risk factor itself, and is associated with the outcome. Multivariable analysis is a method of adjusting for confounders, by including them in the model along with the risk factor (or variable of interest). In our example the age could be considered as a confounder, since length of stay could be influenced by the age of the patient, while age does not influence the injury severity score that could be influenced instead, for example, by the trauma mechanism. From a technical point of view a confounder and a parameter are the same thing, it only varies their interpretation.

7.4 Logistic Regression Models

7.4.1 The Logistic Regression Model

When the outcome variable is not continuous (it can be categorical or binary) the linearity assumption is not fulfilled since there is no linear association between the outcome variable and the predictor. In this case we have to adopt a logistic regression.

Logistic regression explores the association between a categorical outcome variable and one or more explanatory variables; the basic principles are similar to those explained for linear regression. Even in this case the predictors can be continuous, categorical, or binary. If the outcome variable is binary, we would name the regression "binary logistic regression," while if the outcome variable is categorical, the regression would be called "multinomial logistic regression."

From a mathematical point of view (that we will only cite briefly) in the logistic regression model our data are transformed in probability and then in logarithms, obtaining a linear association between the independent variable and the log transformation (or logit) of the outcome variable. After the logit transformation the logistic regression is very similar to a linear regression. Fortunately we do not have to care about these transformations since all statistics software calculate them. The majority of statistics software gives us two effect measures of the logistic regression:

- Coefficient B: is very similar to the beta coefficient of the linear regression, it gives us the measure of the change in logit for each change in the independent variable. Its interpretation is very difficult since it is expressed in a logarithmic scale. For this reason it is always omitted in scientific papers.
- Odd ratio (OR): often expressed also as Exp(B) is the transformation of the coefficient B in an odd ratio. The OR explains the association between the outcome variable and each of the predictors. The measure is a number between 0 and infinity, where the value 1 corresponds to no effect (same odds in the two groups).
  - For binary explanatory variables, the OR is the probability that the outcome variable is present if the explanatory variable is expressed against the probability that the outcome variable is present if the independent variable is absent (see Chap. 8). One of the groups is used as "reference" and the OR will give the increase/decrease in the odds for the corresponding group as compared to the reference group. The reference group for each variable should be clearly stated in the table description. Values between 0 and 1 denote a protective effect of the explanatory variable toward the outcome variable, while values above 1 indicate a positive association between the independent and the dependent variables. For instance, if OR = 2 cases who express the predictor have a twofold increase in the odds of having the outcome variable, as compared to cases who do not express the predictor.
  - For continuous variables the OR represents the increase or decrease in the probability of the outcome event for each increment in the independent variable. An OR > 1 means that for each increment in the independent variable (for example, for each +1 in years of age) the probability of the outcome variable will increment according to the OR. Since continuous variable has a wide range of variable the magnitude of the effect measure is often very reduced, making the interpretation of the real magnitude of the effect less immediate.
  - An alternative way to assess the relationship between a continuous variable and the binary outcome variable is to transform our continuous variable (age) in a grouped (categorical) variable. This transformation is usually adopted to obtain results more immediate and easy to understand with the comparison between several groups. However the choice of the age cut-off is a possible source of bias and it should be taken into account.

The OR should be always reported along with its 95% confidence intervals: for the predictor to be clinically and statistically significant the 95% CI should not cross the value 1. After the 95% CI is reported also the *p*-value for significance test.

7.4.2 Interpreting the Logistic Regression Model: An Example

We now want to study factors associated and related with ICU admission, a binary outcome variable. In this case we have to use a logistic regression. As for the linear regression the first step is to run univariate logistic regressions for each independent variables. The OR we will obtain will be an unadjusted OR, since it comes from an univariate analysis. Let us see Table 7.3 with the example of our trauma dataset:

Table 7.3 Results of the univariate and multiple logistic regression analysis from our example dataset

Independent variable	Dependent variable: ICU admission					
	Univariate logistic regression (unadjusted ORs)			Multiple logistic regression (adjusted ORs)		
	OR	95% CI	*p*-value	OR	95% CI	*p*-value
Sex						
Women (ref)	1	–	–			
Men	2.31	0.65–4.16	0.236	-		
Age	1.11	1.02–1.20	0.012	-		
Age group						
16–30 years (ref)	1	–	–	1		
30–60 years	0.65	0.41–0.80	0.001	0.47	0.12–1.08	0.075
>60 years	21.5	16.1–23.1	0.001	7.65	4.46–9.92	0.001
ISS	1.65	1.2–2.5	0.001	1.74	1.54–2.31	<0.001
Hemodynamic						
Stable (ref)	1	–	–	1		
Shock	14.20	1.25–56.2	0.023	9.89	6.43–12.73	<0.001

Univariate analysis (left side of the table, yellow) shows us that age, injury severity score (ISS), and shock at admission are associated with ICU admission, while sex is not associated with ICU admission. In detail:

- Men have an OR of 2.31 that means that the probability of ICU admission is 2.31 higher compared to women (reference category). However the 95% confidence interval is wide and it crosses the no effect value (value 1); therefore, this result is not significant from a statistical point of view. This is confirmed also by the *p*-value that is >0.05 (*p*-value = 0.236).
- For every increment in the age the probability of ICU admission increment by 1.11 times. This result is statistically significant since the 95% CI does not cross the value 1.
- As an alternative, to evaluate the association between age and ICU admission the age (continuous variable) was grouped and considered as a categorical variable: Age category 1: age 16–30, category 2: age 30–60 and category 3: age > 60. In our example patients with age 30–60 have ~35% lower probability to be admitted in ICU (OR 0.65 95% CI 0.41–0.80) when compared with the chosen reference category (age group 1, 16–30), while patients in >60 years group have a 21.5-fold higher probability when compared with the reference group. This transformation allows us a better understanding of the effect of the age as we see the evident difference with the OR of the age considered as a continuous variable.

- For every increase in the injury severity score the probability of ICU admission increases by 1.65 (95% CI 1.2–2.5). Even there we can notice the significance since the 95% confidence interval does not cross the 1 value.
- Unstable hemodynamics at presentation (shock) is associated with ICU admission with an OR 14.29 (95% CI 1.25–56.2) when compared with stable patients.

The obtained ORs from the univariate analysis are presented as unadjusted odds ratio, i.e. OR not adjusted for potential confounders. In order to evaluate the effect of confounders and evaluate the relationship among the independent variables we have to run multiple logistic regression.

As for the linear regression the choice of the predictors to be included in the model is crucial. Similarly, in order to have a solid model, we have to include in the model a restricted number of covariates (the independent variable): as a rule of thumb, we can include a covariate every ten events in the dependent variable (outcome variable). Another general rule is the choice to include in the model only predictors associated with the outcome variable at the univariate analysis. However the choice of the covariates could be modified (clinical significance at univariate analysis or borderline statistical significance).

In our example we have a very large dataset (<1000 patients) with a large number of events (ICU admission, >150 events). In this case we can run a multiple logistic regression with up to 15 covariates; we therefore will include all the variables associated with ICU admission at the univariate analysis. We must have to notice that we run two univariate analyses for the same variable, the age, once as a continuous variable and once as a categorical variable. In the multiple logistic regression model we will include age only one time. In Table 7.3 the results of the multiple regression are shown on the right side of the table, the pink one. The analysis shows us that age > 60 years, ISS, and shock condition, after adjusting for confounders, are independently related to the ICU admission.

Further Reading[1]

Field A. Discovering statistics using IBM SPSS statistics. 3rd ed. Thousand Oaks, CA: SAGE; 2013.

Sainani KL. Understanding linear regression. PM R. 2013;5(12):1063–8.

Sedgwick P. Simple linear regression. BMJ. 2013;346:f2340.

Sedgwick P. Multiple regression. BMJ. 2013;347:f4373.

Sedgwick P. Logistic regression. BMJ. 2013;347:f4488.

Singh S, Kaplan B, Kim J. Multivariable regression models in clinical transplant research: principles and pitfalls. Transplantation. 2015;99(12):2451–7.

[1]This chapter only provides a brief explanation of the most commonly used statistical regression models. For further readings we would suggest:

Survival Analysis

8

Simone Famularo and Davide Bernasconi

Most of the activities we make in clinical practice have a single, simple aim: fighting the disease to increase survival. Typically, although several medical conditions do not require to face the risk of mortality, the general intellect during the centuries has been captured by the medicine's potential to change the natural history of a disease, tearing a great number of people from a destiny already written. Let us think of cancer, probably the leading cause of death worldwide: in recent years, we made exciting steps forward, changing completely the outcomes for those who are affected. No more than 15 years ago, for example, a diagnosis of metastatic colorectal cancer was a death sentence, while now several therapies and combined approaches are available, reducing sensibly the rate of patients who are condemned. Moreover, the integration of new knowledge derived from molecular medicine, oncology, and surgery is leading us to a new scenario where cancer may become a sort of chronic disease.

Clinical studies play a key role in the continuous development of the treatment of cancer to improve the survival of patients. Thus, a solid knowledge regarding how to collect and analyze survival data is crucial for medical researchers involved in such studies. How can we understand the impact of a treatment in modifying the survival probability of our patients? How can we account for the sequence of events

S. Famularo (✉)
Department of Biomedical Sciences, Humanitas University, Pieve Emanuele, Milan, Italy

Department of Hepatobiliary and General Surgery, IRCCS Humanitas Research Hospital, Rozzano, Milan, Italy

D. Bernasconi
Bicocca Bioinformatics Biostatistics and Bioimaging Centre–B4, School of Medicine and Surgery, University of Milano-Bicocca, Monza, Italy
e-mail: Davide.bernasconi@unimib.it

M. Ceresoli et al. (eds.), *Statistics and Research Methods for Acute Care and General Surgeons*, Hot Topics in Acute Care Surgery and Trauma,
https://doi.org/10.1007/978-3-031-13818-8_8

that occurred at different time points? How can we be sure that an eventual survival benefit is intrinsically connected to the treatment, and not to a more benevolent disease, not so much aggressive? In this chapter, we will focus our attention on these topics through some clinical examples that may better explain how to manage time-to-event data.

8.1 Generalities About Time-to-Event Data

Time-to-event reflects the time elapsed from an initial event (e.g. diagnosis of the disease, surgery, start of treatment) to an event of interest: death, cancer recurrence, a second episode of diverticulitis after conservative treatment, and so on. The event of interest should not be the death in any case: in fact, despite the name commonly used to refer to the statistical methodology, all kinds of events that can occur in a predetermined time-span can be considered in the analysis.

Generally speaking, these techniques are applicable both in randomized clinical trials and in cohort studies (typically prospective but also when data are collected retrospectively).

The most important aspect for the analysis of this type of data is the planned minimum follow-up time of patients. When we set a prospective study, for example, we may plan to enroll patients for 1 year (e.g. at the time they undergo surgery) and to subsequently follow them for further 2 years. The very first patients enrolled at the start of the study will be followed up for almost 3 years, while people enrolled at the end of the study will be followed up for at most 2 years before the study will be closed. Even if we think about a homogeneous cohort of patients sharing very similar treatment and baseline characteristics, it is quite obvious that the probability to observe the event of interest will be different among these two types of patients: let us think about cancer relapse.

The first enrolled patient has been treated and discharged at home, and now we have started the follow-up period: as previously mentioned, our study will last 2 years since end of enrollment, so he has 36 months of time to develop our event of interest, the recurrence. Depending on the type of cancer we are studying, this time period may be enough to observe the event. For the last patient enrolled, however, we will have only 24 months before the study ends to observe the recurrence. This time may also be enough to observe the event but it is much shorter than the follow-up time of the first patient. Both patients may be classified as no-recurrence; however, this may not be because of the treatment we have administered, but because we have observed them for too little time: their recurrence might have occurred when the study was already closed. How can we manage this situation where different follow-up times are present? Moreover, how can we account for the fact that for some patients we may not observe the event of interest (and thus the time of event occurrence)? Should we exclude these patients from our analysis? Obviously not: survival analysis methods have been thought specifically to address these issues, allowing us to manage patients observed for different timespans and that may be still event-free at the end of the study. Another issue that may occur is the patients' drop-out. In fact, a patient may be enrolled in the very early phase of the study, however, for some reason, he may decide to stop his participation in the study before the end of the planned follow-up (he stops to come at the outpatient visits, or he goes to live in another district or country, or simply he changes his mind on the participation at our study). In this latter case, we will have a shorter follow-up, as in the case of those who are enrolled at the end of the study period. For these patients (dropped-out or late enrolment), we surely have an incomplete follow-up. To sum up, we usually have to deal with patients enrolled at different moments and thus with different potential follow-up times who may quit the study before the end. However, as long as the reasons for these differences in the observation time of patients depend only on study logistics and not on the clinical status of patients, we can say the following: for the patients that do not develop the event of interest during the study, we only know that their survival (i.e. event) time is longer than their last observed follow-up: we call these times **censored**.

Box 8.1: What Is Censoring?

Have a look at Fig. 8.1. We have depicted a situation as the last described: in the *Y*-axis, we have the patients enrolled, while in the *X*-axis we have the calendar time. Each patient has a different story: #1 has been enrolled at the study start and has been followed up for the duration of the study without observing a recurrence. Patient #2 has been enrolled on the 4th year and followed up until the end without a recurrence. Patients #3 and #5 have been enrolled at different times, but before the study ended they withdrew: #3 moved to another city and preferred to be followed for his disease in the new location, while #5 did not come to the planned visit, and she did not answer anymore to the phone. Patients #4 and #6 experienced the event of interest (recurrence) at different time points. Thus, since we have observed only two events of interest (patients #4 and #6), our outcome (i.e. the time of event occurrence) is known only for these two subjects. The information we have on the other subjects should not be thrown away! In fact, we have a partial knowledge of the outcome also for censored subjects: we know that their event time is higher than their observed follow-up time. This means that these patients may have a recurrence in the future but we will never observe it. This is true both for patients #1 and #2 who arrived at the end of the study period without experiencing a recurrence as well as for patients #3 who dropped out from the study and patient #5 who was lost to follow-up. Survival analysis methods were designed to account for all these issues, thanks to the following crucial assumption: occurrence of censoring is independent of the likelihood of developing the event of interest. This is certainly true for subject #1 and #2 (the study end is obviously independent from patients survival) and for subject #3 (censoring is due to patient migration so it is again independent from survival), while for patient #5 is not granted: we should speculate what is the reason for loss to follow-up (if the reason is related to the patient status, then independence of censoring assumption may not hold).

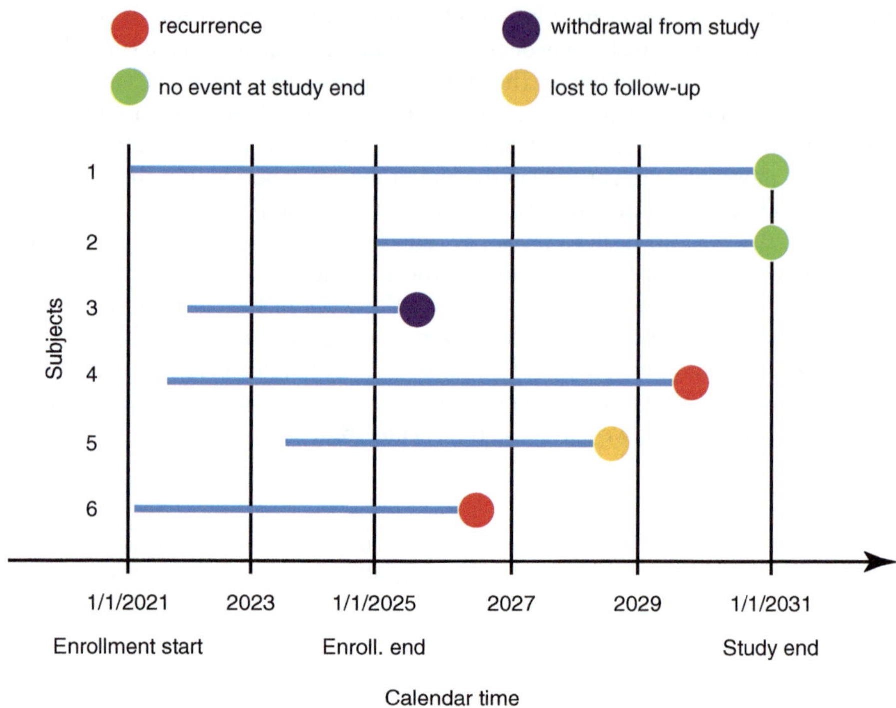

Fig. 8.1 Graphical representation of survival data as they are collected

8.2 The Variables We Need to Make Analysis: Event and Time

Now, we can start to explain how to prepare our data in order to perform a survival analysis. First, for each patient we need a time variable, which should be a continuous variable in which the time (measured in months, days, years, or any other time unit) of observation is expressed. This variable represents the time between the observation start (the first day of a RCT, or the day of surgery, or the day of the diagnosis, depending on the study purpose) and the time of the event or the last time we have notices about the patient. One way to manage this information during data collection is to add two columns in our database, in which we will record the date of the follow-up start, and the date in which the event of interest (e.g. the death) occurred. In case the patient does not experience the event, we will record the last date we have news about him, for example, the date of the last visit. To increase the accuracy and the effectiveness of our analysis, it may be better to have a complete follow-up for all patients: in this sense, it is strongly recommended to update the follow-up at the same time for each patient (this is why, typically, you can find lots of residents that are busy at the phone, making very strange conversation in which they try to gently understand if the patient who has been treated 10 years ago and then has never been seen anymore is still alive or not). When we are making retrospective studies, this could be difficult and challenging and missing data may occur. Recommended methods to manage the missing data (e.g. multiple imputation) are really too advanced for the purpose of this book. A pragmatic solution is to do all the best to find the data: we know about consultants who required their residents to write letters to the registry offices, generating hatred and frustration which ultimately result in abandoning all ambitions of research in the future.

Once we have the two dates, we can simply calculate the difference, in the time unit we prefer, between the two dates, to obtain a continuous variable measuring the time-span and becoming our time variable.

Second, we need for each patient a categorical variable that indicates whether the observed time just calculated represents the time to an event (e.g. death, recurrence, development of a symptom) or to the last follow-up (i.e. censored observation: the patient did not develop the event of interest during the follow-up period). For the analysis we do not need to distinguish among the possible causes for censoring (e.g. study end, loss to follow-up), provided that the independent censoring assumption holds (see the previous paragraph). Thus, this event indicator variable should always be a dichotomous variable (e.g. dead/alive, recurrence/recurrence-free, yes/no). A little recommendation: the event indicator should be coded as a binary variable assuming value 0 for censored observations and value 1 for observed events. This choice is convenient because it corresponds to the default values in many software which will automatically understand this classification. However, some software (such as STATA) always requires to specify which level of the variable indicates who is censored and which level indicates who has the event.

Now our data will look like those represented in Fig. 8.2, while in Fig. 8.3 we can see our toy dataset ready to be loaded into our favorite software to start the analysis.

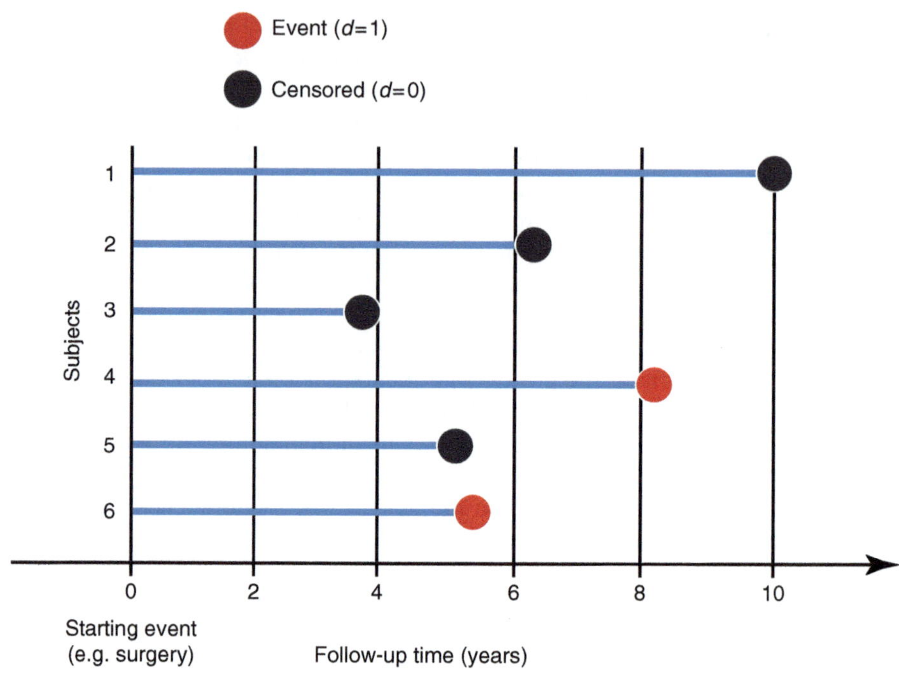

Fig. 8.2 Graphical representation of survival data after they are prepared for being analyzed. The event indicator variable is d and takes value 1 for subjects #4 and #6 who developed an event during follow-up and takes value 0 for the others (censored subjects)

Fig. 8.3 A screenshot of our toy dataset once ready to be analyzed

	A	B	C
1	id	time	event
2	1	10	0
3	2	6.2	0
4	3	3.7	0
5	4	8.3	1
6	5	4.6	0
7	6	4.7	1

8.3 The Survival Curve and Life Tables: The Kaplan–Meier Method

The main goal of survival analysis is to assess the probability that patients from a certain population can survive (or remain event-free) until some time. We want to compute this probability for every time unit (e.g. every year, month, or day) up to a fairly distant time horizon. Once we have prepared the data as mentioned, we can

Table 8.1 Kaplan–Meier estimation of the survival probability over time in our toy dataset

Time index	Time (years)	Number at risk, N_t	Number of deaths, D_t	Number of censored, C_t	Survival probability $S_{t+1} = S_t \times ((N_{t+1} - D_{t+1})/N_{t+1})$
$t = 0$	0	6	0	0	1 (by definition)
$t = 1$	3.7	6	0	1	$1 = 1 \times (6 - 0)/6$
$t = 2$	4.6	5	0	1	$1 = 1 \times (5 - 0)/5$
$t = 3$	4.7	4	1	0	$0.75 = 1 \times (4 - 1)/4$
$t = 4$	6.2	3	0	1	$0.75 = 0.75 \times (3 - 0)/3$
$t = 5$	8.3	2	1	0	$0.375 = 0.75 \times (2 - 1)/2$
$t = 6$	10	1	0	1	$0.375 = 0.75 \times (1 - 0)/1$

proceed to estimate this quantity. The result will typically be presented as a survival curve, in which the *X*-axis shows the follow-up time, and the *Y*-axis the probability to survive (the proportion of people surviving) until that moment.

The estimation of the survival probability used to generate the curve is typically done using the Kaplan–Meier method, which can be described by the following formula:

$$S_{t+1} = S_t \times \left(\left(N_{t+1} - D_{t+1} \right) / N_{t+1} \right)$$

This means that if we know the survival at time t (S_t) we can compute the survival at next time $t + 1$ (S_{t+1}) by multiplying S_t with the probability of surviving in the next time unit $t + 1$. The last one is computed as the proportion of patients NOT died at $t + 1$ (i.e. patients alive at $t + 1$ minus patients died at $t + 1$: $N_{t+1} - D_{t+1}$) over patients alive at $t + 1$ (N_{t+1}). The first value of the survival S_0 is by definition equal to 1 since at time 0 all patients are alive. How does the method account for censored subjects? At time $t + 1$ the number of subjects still alive is obtained by taking patients alive at t (N_t) and subtracting patients who died at t (D_t) but also subjects censored at t (C_t), thus $N_{t+1} = N_t - D_t - C_t$.

With this formula, we can create a table like the following (Table 8.1):

In the first column only times when something happens (i.e. at least one patient died or censored) are reported in increasing order. The number at risk reported in the second column represents the patients that have not yet experienced the event of interest at that time point and that have not yet been censored. This number will decrease as time passes and give us a very important piece of information regarding how reliable the survival estimate is (see Box 8.2 to better understand why this is very important). In the third column, we find the number of deaths: in this example, we are measuring the overall survival but in other examples here we can find the number of patients who experienced the event of interest, at the time it occurred. Then we have a column for censored observations. Finally, for all the relevant time points, the survival probability is computed. As time increases, the value of the survival can only remain the same or decrease and the value is updated only at times when at least one patient has the event (for this reason, the plotted curve has a "stair" shape). To know the estimated survival probability at a certain time (e.g. 5 years), we need to find in the time column the maximum time lower than the time of interest and read the corresponding survival value. For instance, the estimated survival at 5 years is 0.75 (we should look at the row where time = 4.7).

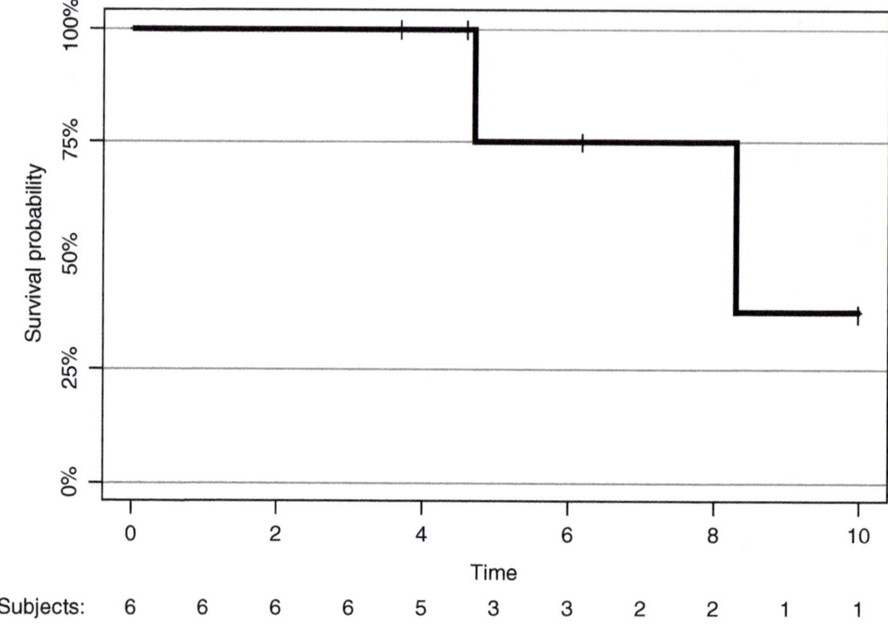

Fig. 8.4 Kaplan–Meier survival curve estimated on toy data

Looking at Fig. 8.4, we can easily understand the survival probability of our cohort at different time points. Finding the intersection among *X* and *Y* axis, we can estimate that after 5 years of follow-up, 75% of our patients are survivors. By definition, to estimate the median survival of our cohort, we need to follow the *Y*-axis at 0.50 and find the intersection on the *X*-axis: in this example, the median survival time of our cohort is a bit higher than 8 years. As expected, patients are 100% alive at time 0 (the *X*-axis origin): this obvious assumption conditions the figure of the curve, which is always decreasing to the right, that is the direction in which the time increases. The slower the curve decreases, the higher will be the survival of patients, even after a long time. When the curve decreases sharply, we are facing a disease that is very aggressive, with a high probability of death. When we compare two survival curves, for example, estimated on two groups of patients under two different treatments, the higher one will belong to the treatment with the best prognosis (we will reconsider this theme after).

We can also provide information about the censoring: a proper figure, in fact, should report the presence of patients censored at each time point. This is usually visualized by a sign on the curve (in our example, a small vertical line is present when there is a censored case). Remember that the aim of your graphic representation is not to hide data, but to summarize the highest quantity of information and to make it easy to be understood by other physicians. Depending on the sample size, the survival curve can be more of a staircase rather than a proper curve: the higher the number of patients, the more the survival line becomes similar to a smooth curve.

Another consideration should be made about the direction of the curve which can provide a description of the natural history of a disease. For example, if the survival curve tends to flatten after a certain time point, this suggests that patients who are still event-free at that time point are not anymore at risk of developing the event. In contrast, if the curve falls down to zero this means that after the time the curve reaches the horizontal axis no patient survives.

Be careful about extrapolating the results of a curve beyond a certain time point! The Kaplan–Meier curve could be artificially projected up to very far time points that we do not really observe. For example, one could be tempted to draw the survival curve until 15 years, even if patients in the cohort were observed for a maximum of 5 years. This is very speculative and should be avoided. A good practice is to report the median follow-up time of the study (together with inter-quartile range), allowing readers to know which survival times have been really observed (see Box 8.2 to know how to calculate appropriately the median follow-up time of your study).

Box 8.2: Patient-At-Risk and Median Follow-Up Time: How to Interpret

We now want to focus our attention on two important aspects both connected to the correct interpretation of a survival curve: the number of patients at risk in the right tail of the curve and the calculation of the median follow-up time.

All statistical estimators are subject to some variability which reflects our uncertainty on the point estimate we calculate and this variability depends also on the inverse of the sample size: the higher is the number of subjects on which the estimate is calculated, the lower is our uncertainty around that value. This is true also for Kaplan–Meier curves with one additional caveat: the sample size decreases through time. The number of patients at risk is in fact eroded for two reasons: patients who die (or have the event of interest) and patients who are censored. As a consequence, even if our initial sample size is particularly high, as we move towards the right tail of the curve the number of patients at risk becomes smaller and smaller. This means that also the precision of our Kaplan–Meier survival estimates decreases through time and, from a certain time onwards, may become unreliable because its updated value could be based on a very small number of patients still at risk. In Fig. 8.5 we show a Kaplan–Meier curve together with 95% confidence interval (shaded area). As you can see, the amplitude of the confidence interval increases through time suggesting that the estimate becomes less and less precise. At time 4.5 we have only 10 patients still at risk: the curve is thus updated based on the mortality observed on that restricted group of patients. Reading survival probability estimates on the right tail of the curve must be considered with caution.

Providing a summary measure of follow-up time is always requested when reporting the results of a cohort study. A typical measure is the median which can be easily calculated directly on the observed follow-up time of patients. However, with survival times we may get in trouble even for this simple task. In fact, if our end-point is death or if our observation ends as patients experience the event of interest, simply calculating the median of the observed times would lead to an underestimation of the follow-up time. The survival time of patients who died is obviously shorter than their potential follow-up time (especially for those who died early). The question is: for how long would we have followed patients if they did not die? How can we obtain a more accurate estimate of this quantity? Surprisingly, the solution is again Kaplan–Meier but… reversed! In this case, censored times are those we are really interested in, while survival times represent a lower limit for the true follow-up time of a patient; thus, we can simply estimate the curve considering censored observation as events and death as censorings (Fig. 8.6). The time where this curve reaches 50% is about 4.2 and this is the best estimate of the median follow-up time we can get. On the same data, if we calculated the simple median of the observed times, we would get 1.55, a clear underestimation.

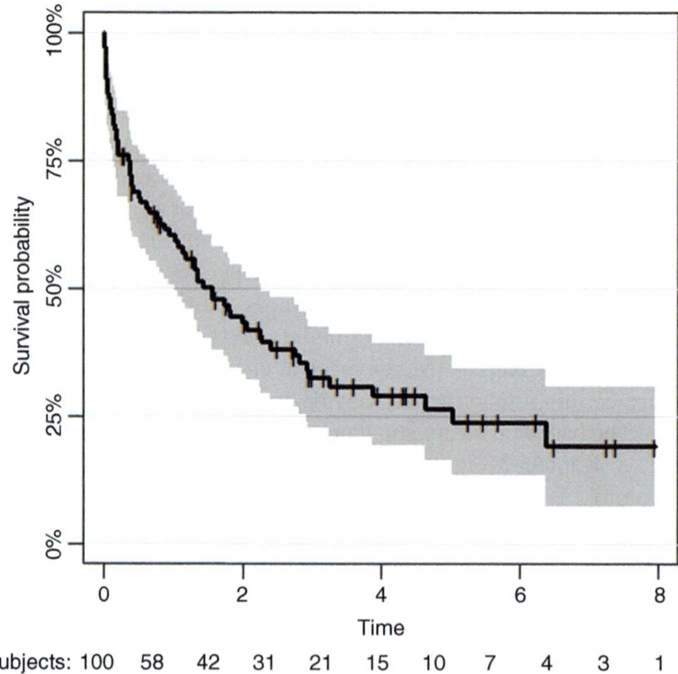

Fig. 8.5 Kaplan–Meier survival curve with 95% confidence interval (shaded area) on a made-up dataset

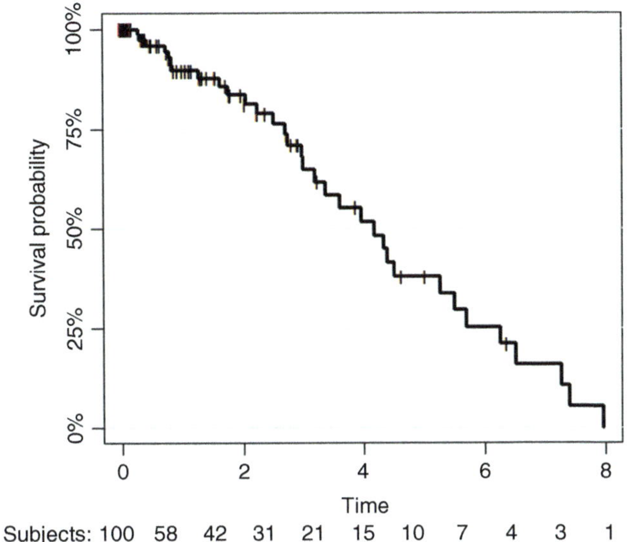

Fig. 8.6 Reverse Kaplan–Meier applied to the same data of Fig. 8.5. Events and censored observations are flipped over

Example Box: Part 1

DISCLOSURE: The following data are completely created, and the results obtained do not depict a real scenario. The example is completely invented, and the conclusion does not want to suggest anything. The comparisons are made reliable to better highlight the management a clinician should employ to make survival analysis; however, the setting and all the data are not taken from reality.

We are surgical oncologists, and after a few years we have started a laparoscopic program to treat HCC patients. We would like to know if the long-term survival of those patients treated by laparoscopy is longer, similar, or shorter than the classical open approach. For this purpose, we decide to set up a retrospective study, to compare the overall survival among the two surgical approaches.

We know from the literature and the guidelines that the overall survival for liver tumors is conditioned not only by the surgical technique but also by the tumor burden (number and size of the nodules), the comorbidities and the age of patients, their underlying liver function, and some histological characteristics: since the retrospective nature of the study, we want to collect all this information to adjust the risk and be sure about the treatment effect on survival. We start to create a data-sheet in Excel where we collect all the data we need to make our analysis. Likewise, we decide to collect all the following variables: patient's ID, age (continuous variable, years), sex (categorical variables, levels: male and female), number of nodules (continuous variable), size of the nodules (continuous variable, cm), presence of cirrhosis (categorical variable, levels: yes and no), MELD score (continuous variable), HBV or HCV infections (categorical variables, levels: yes or not), type of procedure executed (categorical variable, levels: open, laparoscopy), date of the procedure, presence of microvascular invasion (categorical variable, levels: yes and no), and satellitosis (categorical variable, levels: yes and no). To simplify the software job, we transform all the categorical variables in no = 0 and yes = 1, female = 0 and male = 1. After this, we also need to collect the variables we need for survival analysis: the event status (alive or dead) and the follow-up time. Since our primary end-point is overall survival, we start checking in our hospital management software all the last visits of our patients, to know if our enrolled patients are still alive or not at the present date. In case we did not visit the patient recently, we decide to call by phone number to speak directly with the patients or the parents to know about their follow-up. We want to know their status at the present day, so we create a column in which we insert the date of the last contact (if the patient is alive) or the death date. Although we want to do the maximum to find the most updated news about the patients' follow-up, for a few of them we won't be able to have any news after a certain period: to don't lose patients, we decide to insert the date of the last available contact, with the event status at that time. Those patients will be considered as censored, but they will still contribute to our analysis, although differently if compared with patients with completed follow-up.

To create our time variable (called OS in this study), we simply make a subtraction between the date of surgery and the date of last follow-up or the date of death (see Fig. 8.7).

After this screening, between 2008 and 2020 we have enrolled 464 patients treated by surgery in our center for HCC. Of them, 65 (14.0%) have been treated by laparoscopy. On a first look, we know that 301 patients (64.8%) died during the follow-up period, 294 in the open surgery group, and 7 in the laparoscopy one. Now we would like to know if this difference is significant and if there is an overall survival advantage with one technique or not.

	A	B	C	D	E	F	G	H	I	J	K	L	M	N	O	P
1	ID	Age	Sex	Cirrhosis	MELD	HCV	HBV	N_nodules	Size_nodules	date_of_surgery	Laparoscopy	microvascular_invasion	satellitosis	death_event	date of last contact/date of dead	OS
2	2005033951	57	0	1	14	0	0	1	2	06/07/2005	0	0	0	1	03/12/2012	89.04605263
3	2005040387	63	0	1	6	0	0	1	1.6	05/07/2005	0	1	0	0	12/08/2021	138.0592105
4	2005047733	44	1	1	6	0	1	1	2	09/09/2005	1	0	0	0	12/08/2021	136.9078947
5	2005051308	58	1	1	7	1	1	1	1.3	29/09/2005	0	1	0	1	11/07/2014	105.4934211
6	2006060873	56	0	1	11	1	0	1	1.5	06/12/2006	1	0	0	1	25/04/2008	16.64473684
7	2007013647	71	0	0	5	1	0	1	2	26/01/2007	1	0	0	0	12/08/2021	119.3092105
8	2007029838	64	0	1	7	1	0	1	2	10/05/2007	0	0	0	0	12/08/2021	69.80263158
9	2007034838	47	0	1	6	0	1	1	1.5	08/06/2007	0	0	0	0	12/08/2021	71.34868421
10	2008010513	58	0	1	7	0	1	1	1.5	07/01/2008	1	1	1	1	01/06/2010	28.81578947
11	2008017967	56	0	1	11	0	1	1	2	26/02/2008	1	0	0	1	24/04/2012	49.96710526
12	2008022038	66	1	1	6	1	0	1	1.8	18/03/2008	1	0	1	0	12/08/2021	105.5921053
13	2008030565	75	0	0	6	0	0	1	1.6	20/05/2008	0	0	0	0	12/08/2021	103.5197368
14	2008042122	62	0	1	11	0	0	1	1.8	08/08/2008	0	1	1	1	22/09/2016	97.59868421
15																

Fig. 8.7 An example of a dataset managed with one of the most popular software. All the variables appear as number (and no free text), with only one data per each cell

8.4 Comparing Survival Curves: The Log-Rank Test

During our clinical research, most of the time we are more interested in comparing the effect of two (or more) treatments on survival, rather than knowing the survival of the whole cohort. The Kaplan–Meier estimator can simply be applied separately to groups defined by a categorical variable to evaluate the survival probability (as well as the median survival) observed in each group (provided that enough patients are present in all groups). For example, in a clinical trial with a survival outcome, we might be interested in comparing survival between participants receiving a new drug as compared to a placebo (or standard therapy). In an observational study, we might be interested in comparing survival between men and women, or between persons with and without a particular risk factor (e.g. hypertension or diabetes). However, rather than simply looking at the curves observed in the samples, one might also be interested in assessing the association of treatment or another variable with survival using a statistical hypothesis test.

Facing this issue could seem very simple, after all the knowledge acquired in the previous chapters of this book. In fact, once we know the total number of deaths for each treatment, we could imagine simply making a Chi-square test to compare the proportion of events among the groups. Another approach that we could regard as feasible after reading this book may be to perform a *T* test to compare the mean of time-to-event among groups. Both the ideas are wrong. Let us think again to the first paragraph of this chapter: when we face survival data, we have several issues: patients are observed for different periods, the event of interest can be observed during the follow-up time or occur later, and finally patients may not have completed the predetermined follow-up time. In a few words: we need to account for censoring! Censored observations carry information that we do not want to lose. The log-rank test was designed to tackle these issues, providing us a tool that accounts for the occurrence of events in time and for censoring. There are other types of procedures we can employ to test the hypothesis of equal survival among groups; however, in this chapter we will discuss only the log-rank test, which is undoubtedly the most popular in clinical applications.

The log-rank test considers the null hypothesis (H_0) of equal survival between two or more independent populations. In other words, the test helps to judge whether the survival curves we observe on the sample groups are compatible with the possibility that the "true" survival curves (i.e. the curves in the whole populations of interest from which samples are drawn) are identical (overlapping) between groups or not. The log-rank test is actually a particular kind of stratified chi-square test as it compares observed vs. expected numbers of events at each time point over the follow-up period (the stratification variable is time). Analogously to the other statistical tests, we simply obtain a *p*-value which should be compared with the chosen level of significance to assess whether the treatment groups are significantly different or not in terms of survival. If we are comparing more than two treatments, it may be useful to make several pairwise log-rank test, which means comparing the treatments one-by-one: this will provide us a better explanation of where the differences are, because, for example, two treatments could have similar survival probability, but different from a third treatment. Some correction of the *p*-value (e.g. Bonferroni or more advanced methods) should then be applied to account for the multiple testing problem (similarly to what is done, for example, by ANOVA post-hoc tests).

Box 8.3: OS, DFS, RFS: Defining the Outcomes

A clear definition of the end-point of interest is fundamental, and this is why in the methodology section of research papers, it is mandatory to specify this aspect. Here we provide for you some standard definition of the most popular end-points in surgical oncology, for your convenience.

- Overall survival (OS): The time from the date of treatment (surgery, drug delivery, etc.) to the date of any cause of death.
- Disease free survival (DFS): The time from the date of treatment to the date of the first event among death for any cause or recurrence of the tumor. Consequently, this is a combined end-point that considers together both types of "failures", deaths and recurrence. This is also sometimes called recurrence-free survival (RFS).
- Time to recurrence (TTR): The time from the date of treatment to the date of recurrence after the treatment. In this case, patients who died during the follow-up are censored at the date of death or, perhaps more properly, death is considered as a "competing risk" (this would require ad hoc analytical methods rather than Kaplan–Meier and log-rank test).

However, be aware that these terms can be used to refer to slightly different end-points. So, besides names you may want to use for your end-points, it is highly recommended to always report each event of interest you included in the analysis.

Example Box: Part 2

Now we have prepared our data, and we want to compare survival among the two surgical groups. We launch our statistical software (we can use, for example, *R*, version 4.0.6) and we upload the database. First, we calculate the median follow-up time, using the reverse Kaplan–Meier method: in our cohort, the median FU was 69.93 months (IQR 39.44–110.10).

Then, we launch a Kaplan–Meier. Here below is the life table obtained (we kept only the rows of 12, 36, and 60 months).

Laparoscopy = No						
Time	N. risk	N. event	Survival	Std. err	Lower 95% CI	Upper 95% CI
12	322	70	0.823	0.0192	0.786	0.861
36	211	83	0.599	0.0252	0.552	0.651
60	124	47	0.448	0.0270	0.398	0.504

Laparoscopy = Yes						
Time	N. risk	N. event	Survival	Std. err	Lower 95% CI	Upper 95% CI
12	51	2	0.965	0.0241	0.919	1.000
36	14	5	0.822	0.0646	0.705	0.959
60	5	0	0.822	0.0646	0.705	0.959

Then we create a survival curve, where we also insert the *p*-value obtained by the log-rank test (when you create these figures, it is always recommendable to add the *p*-value).

If we focus on the survival curve, we can immediately understand the survival differences between the two treatments. At the bottom left, we visualize the *p*-value obtained by the log-rank test. As commonly a $p < 0.05$ is accepted for significance, here the two treatments are significantly different, and laparoscopy (the light blue line) is superior to open surgery (the red line) in terms of overall survival. In our sample, we can conclude that the two treatments are different observing the curves, which showed a large spread between each other. In fact, the spread among the two curves indicates the effect of treatment on survival in our sample, allowing to visualize how "large" is the difference (Fig. 8.8). The figure can give us other important information The little crosses on the two survival curves are the censored patients: the density on the curve of the crosses gives us information about how many patients we have followed for all the period. Another important information derives from the table "number at risk": in fact, patients in the laparoscopic group are few, and approximately after 30 months of observation, the survival curve becomes flattened, with only some crosses on it. This means that no death event has been recorded in that group after that time, and the reduction of the number of patients at risk is conditioned by the censoring. When there is so little data, we should carefully evaluate the meaning of those results at least at that specific time points: it is unrealistic that those who were treated by laparoscopy stop to die at a certain time point. Probably, enlarging the sample size, and completing the follow-up, we will note other death events that could better represent the real survival tendency of these patients. Thus, always carefully consider the table of number at risk, because it can give you important information on how realistic the survival prediction is, particularly far in time.

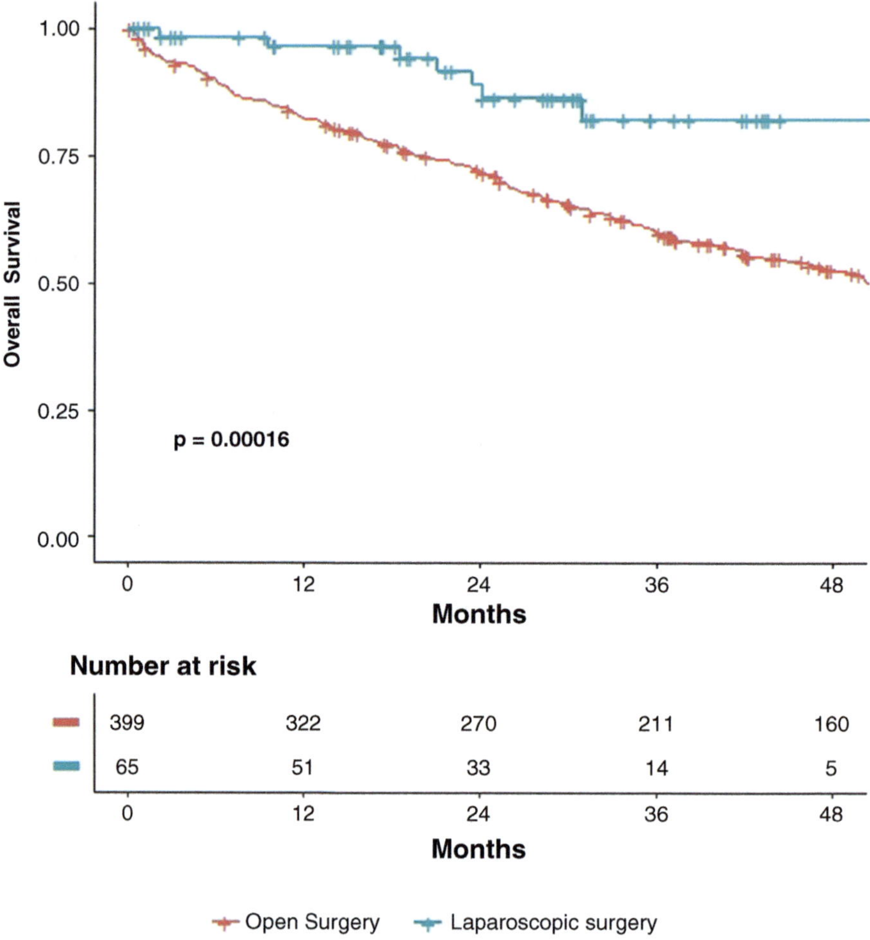

Fig. 8.8 Kaplan–Meier curves and log-rank test *p*-value of overall survival between surgical techniques

8.5 A Regression Model to Assess the Association of Multiple Predictors with a Survival Outcome: The Cox "Proportional Hazards" Model

The comparison of survival curves between two (or more) treatments is a sort of univariate survival analysis, in which we assess the association of a single risk factor (the treatment) with the outcome. However, we may desire to study several factors simultaneously, as when we perform linear or logistic regressions. We need a regression model, suitable for time-to-event data, that allows us to assess independently the impact of a risk factor in the occurrence of the event of interest in time and consequently to assess if the effect we may have recognized with the Kaplan–Meier method is real or is driven by some other factors (possible confounders). However, directly modeling the survival function is statistically challenging (although some possible solutions have been proposed). It turns out that it is much more convenient to focus on another quantity of time called "hazard rate." This can be viewed as an "instantaneous velocity" of the event occurrence at each time or, in other words, as the risk for a patient alive at a certain time to develop the event in the next instant.

One of the most popular regression methods in survival analysis is the Cox proportional hazards model. It is composed of two parts which are multiplied together: one is the "baseline hazard," the hazard of patients with reference level of all covariates; the other is the effect of each covariate on the baseline hazard, showing how the hazard modifies when covariates change. The first part can be difficult to estimate properly (although suitable estimators have been proposed) but what we really care about is the second part: Sir David Cox invented a method to estimate the effect of covariates without taking care of the baseline hazard (that is why this method is still so popular!). In the end, in a Cox model, the measure of effect is the hazard ratio (HR), which tells us how many times we have to multiply the baseline hazard to obtain the hazard of another level of a covariate. For example, if the HR between treatment A and B is 2, this means that patients treated with A develop the event two times faster than patients treated with B. We can also say that the HR between B and A is 0.5, meaning that the velocity of occurrence of the event is halved for patients treated with B with respect to those treated with A. People tend to interpret HR as a risk ratio (similarly to what happens for the odds ratio). This is not totally correct as we should always bear in mind that the hazard is not a simple risk but a sort of "risk in time." However, as with risk ratio and odds ratio, an HR approaching 1 suggests no effect of that covariate, an HR > 1 means that the covariate is probably a risk factor and an HR < 1 indicates a protective role.

Another analogy with risk ratio and odds ratio is that also HR is usually shown with its (95%) confidence interval and possibly the *p*-value. A statistically significant effect is considered when the confidence interval does not include 1 (the null value) or when the *p*-value is lower than a nominal level (typically 5%). Beyond statistical significance it is always important to look also at the clinical relevance of the estimated effect, especially in observational studies where no a priori sample size calculations were made.

Have a look at Table 8.2:

Table 8.2 Cox regression analysis

		95% CI		
	HR	Lower limit	Upper limit	*p*
Age > =75 (versus <75)	1.012	0.990	1.034	0.282
Charlson comorbidity index (per unit)	1.040	0.905	1.195	0.581
Presence of cirrhosis (versus not)	1.966	1.161	3.328	0.012
Number of nodules (per unit)	1.151	0.815	1.627	0.424
Microvascular invasion (versus not)	1.830	1.202	2.786	0.005
Post-operative complication (versus not)	1.221	0.736	2.023	0.440
Laparoscopy (vs. open approach)	0.754	0.654	0.987	0.043
Post-op liver complication (versus not)	2.524	1.344	4.739	0.004

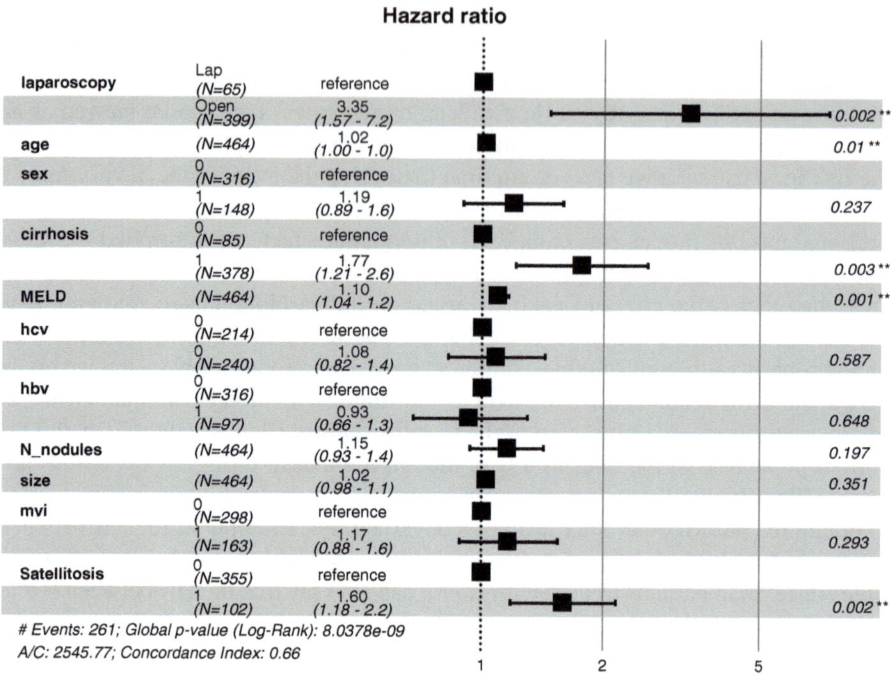

Fig. 8.9 Forest plot depicting the results of a multivariate Cox regression as per our example

This is how to report the results of a Cox regression in a table. You will notice that each variable is followed by brackets, which contain the reference value against which the level of interest of each covariate was compared. It is very important to always declare what we are comparing! The width of the CI is a measure of precision of our estimates: the sharper the CI is, the more precise the obtained estimate is. As already said, the HR may take values from 1 to infinity for risk factors or may take a decimal value between 0 and 1 for protective factors.

To make things clearer, just have a look at one of the variables, e.g. post-op liver complication: the HR is 2.524, 95% CI: 1.344–4.739, $p = 0.004$.

In this example, we expect that experiencing a post-operative liver complication increases the hazard of death by 2.54-fold when compared with patients who did not experience such complications. The result is statistically significant because 1 is not included in the confidence interval, as evident also by the p-value that is <0.05. In case we are analyzing a continuous variable, the interpretation of the HR is slightly different: the HR represents the multiplicative factor of the hazard for a 1 unit increase in our covariate. In our example, the number of tumor nodules has an HR of 1.151: this means that we expect that the hazard increases by a factor of 1.151 for each additional nodule (the result is not statistically significant). Remember also that, as with other regression tools, we should also explore the assumption of linearity in the effect of continuous covariates (we cannot hereby explain this issue in detail.

To calculate the "excess of hazard" caused by a factor, we may subtract 1 to the HR (HR-1) and then multiply the result per 100. For example, when microvascular invasion is present, we expect the hazard of patients without this problem to increase by 83% (thus, to almost double). In case the HR is below 1, we need to remember to invert the subtraction (1-HR). For example, laparoscopy is associated with a hazard decrease of 25% with respect to patients treated with open surgery.

Another consideration should be made about the number of variables we can insert in a Cox regression. This is a very tricky issue; however, a very simple rule to take home is the so-called one to ten rule: to create a reliable model with valid parameter estimates, we can add an explanatory variable for every ten events that occurred in our cohort. So, if we are investigating the risk of mortality and in our cohort we observe 56 events, we may simultaneously include no more than five to six covariates in our model.

A final consideration should be made to clarify one important limit of the Cox regression. This technique relies on a crucial assumption: the hazard proportionality assumption. Namely, Cox model assumes that the hazards in levels of each covariate (for example, between treatment A and B) are proportional over time, which implies that the effect of a risk factor should be constant over time. So, if HR of A vs. B is 2 we are assuming that patients treated with A die twice more quickly than those treated with B at the beginning of the follow-up, as well as after some time, till the end of follow-up. This assumption is not always tenable as some treatments may have an early efficacy which is lost during time or may show only a late efficacy. We can verify this assumption by several tools, using statistical tests, or graphically. One of the most popular methods is based on scaled Schoenfeld residuals. Otherwise, we can try to figure out whether the assumption may hold directly by looking at the survival curves obtained with the Kaplan–Meier method: if the curves of the two treatments cross each other, then the assumption is definitively violated. This suggests that the hazards are not proportional over time, and the Cox regression is not appropriate: some adjustment must be made to account for non-proportionality. One simple approach is to run a stratified Cox model for the variable for which the assumption is violated (again, refer to more advanced references for details).

Example Box: Part 3—Estimating the Association of Many Variables with Mortality

To complete our survival analysis, we would be sure that the survival advantage we have recorded for laparoscopic patients is not linked to other factors that could have justified the significant difference observed. For example, the laparoscopic advantage may be driven by the fact that patients submitted to laparoscopy presented themselves with a more favorable disease, more little, with a reduced number of nodules, less patient's comorbidities, younger age, or whatever other medical reason that could modify the risk of mortality.

Moreover, now we know that a laparoscopic approach may increase survival, but we would like to quantify how much the risk is modified when compared with the open technique.

In this condition, we definitely need to perform a multiple Cox Regression analysis. There are several ways to decide which variables should be inserted in the multivariate model, but this is not the point of this paragraph. We will run a model with all the confounders we have at disposal in our dataset. Just note that the total number of deaths is 301, so following the "one to ten" rule of thumbs we can insert in the model up to 30 variables: such a great number of confounders can be explored with this cohort!

As a result of the Cox regression (Fig. 8.9), we can now estimate that performing an open approach independently increases the hazard of mortality by 235% (HR 3.35, 95% CI: 1.5–7.2, *p*: 0.002) when compared to the laparoscopic one, fixing all the other confounders we have investigated. This is a strong confirmation of the effect of the treatment because now we could be sure that, at least for all the variables investigated (remember that, particularly in the retrospective studies, there could be always other confounders that we did not record that could justify the risk variation), there is an independent and significant survival difference linked to the treatment we are investigating. There are also other factors that, alone and independently, modify the hazard of mortality according to our analysis: the age (an increase of mortality by 2% per each year), the presence of cirrhosis, the MELD score (10% of increase per each point of MELD), and the presence of satellitosis. Now we can conclude satisfactorily our survival analysis and we can discuss the results we have measured!

Meta-Analysis

9

Marco Ceresoli, Fikri M. Abu-Zidan, and Federico Coccolini

9.1 Introduction

Meta-analysis is one of the cornerstones of evidence-based medicine. A meta-analysis is a statistical method allowing to combine the results of two or more studies, giving a pooled estimate result as much closer as possible to the truth, trying to minimize errors. Moreover, the meta-analysis allows to identify differences among the results of the included studies [1].

The rationale to perform meta-analysis is the possibility to collect the results of all the existing studies on a topic and to combine them in a more precise and powerful statistical analysis, based on a higher sample size.

Several types of research data can be analyzed using meta-analysis like comparing an intervention versus another intervention or multiple interventions (randomized controlled studies or case–control studies), results of diagnostic studies, and prognostic data.

Generally meta-analysis is used to combine results of randomized controlled trials, giving the highest level of evidence available, according to the principles of the evidence-based medicine; however, since meta-analysis is only a statistical method,

M. Ceresoli (✉)
General and Emergency Surgery Department, School of Medicine and Surgery,
Milano-Bicocca University, Monza, Italy
e-mail: marco.ceresoli@unimib.it

F. M. Abu-Zidan
The Research Office, College of Medicine and Health Science,
United Arab Emirates University, Al Ain, United Arab Emirates

F. Coccolini
Department of General, Emergency and Trauma Surgery, Pisa University Hospital, Pisa, Italy

M. Ceresoli et al. (eds.), *Statistics and Research Methods for Acute Care and General Surgeons*, Hot Topics in Acute Care Surgery and Trauma,
https://doi.org/10.1007/978-3-031-13818-8_9

it can also be used to combine results of non-randomized studies: in that case the level of evidence of the obtained results is lower. The present chapter describes the fundamental steps needed to (1) perform a meta-analysis and to (2) critically appraise a meta-analysis study.

9.2 The Question

The first step is the definition of the question: This is the fundamental node. The question should follow the PICO model, according to the principles of evidence-based medicine [2]: This stands for (1) P: patients/population, who are the patients or population that you will study? (2) I: intervention: what is the intervention that you are studying? (3) C: control: what is your control? (4) O: outcomes, what are your outcome variables?. This acronym reassumes the fundamental characteristics that a good question should have: a clear definition of the *patients/population* (the disease, for example) in which the investigated *intervention* is compared with a defined *control* for a specific *outcome.*

Once the question is well defined, then the further steps will be a systematic search of the literature with retrieval of all eligible studies, the evaluation of the quality of the studies, and data extraction from each included study. The results of the studies can be pooled and the result of the meta-analysis can be demonstrated by a forest plot.

In this chapter we will use a hypothetical meta-analysis and we will follow it through all the steps. Data are completely invented. Our question is the comparison of laparoscopic appendectomy (intervention) versus open appendectomy (control) in adult patients with acute appendicitis (patients) in postoperative complications and operative time (outcomes). The first step will be the systematic review of the literature.

9.3 Systematic Review of the Literature

A systematic review of the literature is an essential prerequisite before performing the meta-analysis. Once the PICO question is clear, a fundamental step is to define which databases and resources to systematically search and the inclusion and exclusion criteria of these studies. Defining the search protocol with the help of a search methodologist (expert librarian) before starting the systematic review helps to be able to reproduce the results. An inaccurate literature review, without a clear protocol that finds all available relevant data, will lead to biased results. This could happen as a result of an inaccurate review or for the inclusion of "cherry-picked" studies to support a personal viewpoint. For example, if we exclude (accidentally or deliberately) some large sample studies with negative results, we may have a pooled estimate effect influenced by our selection bias. The search, exclusion, and selection process should be described in detail and shown in a flow chart diagram, as recommended by the PRISMA guidelines [3] (Fig. 9.1).

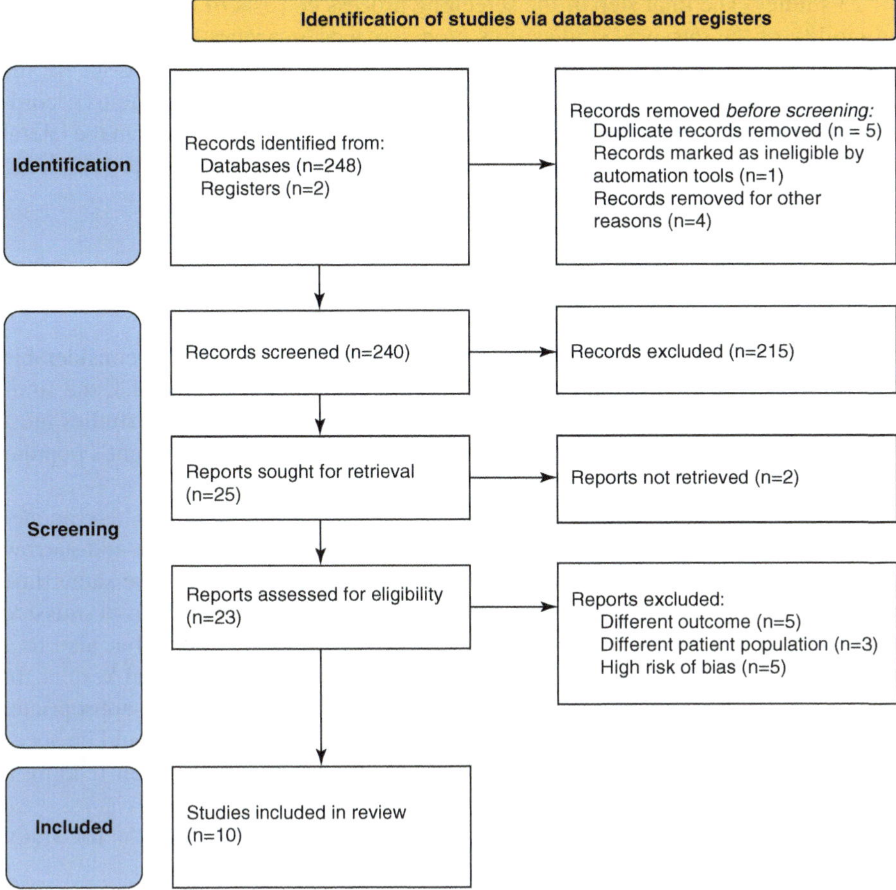

Fig. 9.1 An example of the PRISMA flow diagram

Let us look at our hypothetical example. The flow diagram describes our reviewing process.

The first level contains information about the identifications of studies addressing our topic, based on the criteria adopted and described in the methods section.

The first box describes the number of retrieved records, and the right lateral box contains the number of excluded articles before the screening: we retrieved a total of 250 studies and 10 were initially excluded because duplicate records or other reasons (for example, a study written not in English).

The second level contains information about the screening process and its steps.

The first box describes the first screening (generally made with title and abstract analysis: **Titles are first screened and then those of interest have their abstracts screened**) with the indication of the number of excluded studies and reports indicated in the lateral box: among the remaining 240 studies after a screening of title and abstract 215 were excluded. Two more records were not available giving a total of 23 studies. The final step of the screening process consists of the assessment for eligibility of the retrieved studies: this process needs an accurate evaluation of the full text of each study; if a study is excluded, we must indicate the reasons for the exclusion. Among the remaining 23 studies we excluded another 13 studies according to the chosen criteria and we indicated the reasons for the exclusion in the lateral box (and in the results section of the meta-analysis). Finally, we have the remaining 10 studies that will be included in the analysis.

9.4 Meta-analysis Appropriateness: Study Inclusion

Another important requirement for a meta-analysis is the absence of considerable clinical or methodological heterogeneity among the selected studies, i.e. the similarity of study design, treatments, and outcomes. Ideally all included studies must have the same design, the same treatment investigated in the same patient's population, and the same endpoint.

There are no statistical tests that could assess and measure clinical heterogeneity and great attention should be given to its description: too precise and narrow inclusion criteria will reduce heterogeneity to the minimum but at the same time they may lead to exclusion of some important studies; conversely, too permissive inclusion criteria will lead to a greater number of included studies but also to a higher clinical or methodological heterogeneity with possible biased results. In case of great clinical heterogeneity, a meta-analysis will not be appropriate. Inclusion and exclusion criteria (on which heterogeneity depends) should be accurately described; You should give great attention to this section when reading a meta-analysis!

Here are some examples of clinical heterogeneity not appropriate for study inclusion:

- the inclusion of a study comparing laparoscopic appendectomy (intervention) versus robotic appendectomy in patients with acute appendicitis when other studies have open appendectomy as the control group.
- the inclusion of a study comparing laparoscopic appendectomy (intervention) versus open appendectomy (control) in only pediatric patients with acute appendicitis (different population) when the other studies evaluate adults.
- the inclusion of a retrospective study comparing laparoscopic appendectomy (intervention) versus open appendectomy (control) in patients with acute appendicitis (population) when the other studies are randomized trials.

9.5 Study Quality Assessment and the Risk of Bias

During the process of studies' evaluation and inclusion in the meta-analysis, it is very important to assess the study quality and the possible risk of bias (see Chap. 4). The presence of bias may under- or overestimate the value of the outcome. Since the conclusions and the interpretation of the results of a meta-analysis depend on the results of the included studies, the presence of biased results of a single included study especially with large sample may lead to misleading conclusions. Therefore, for each included study, the possible presence of biases should be carefully assessed and described. Several tools and scales have been developed for this purpose.

For **randomized trials**, the Cochrane collaboration developed a specific tool for bias risk assessment [1]. This tool evaluates six specific domains containing all possible sources of biases and evaluates the risk of bias in three levels: low risk, some concerns, and high risk.

The six domains are:

- Bias arising from the randomization process: This domain evaluates if the allocation sequence is random and adequately concealed and if there are differences between the characteristics of the randomized groups.
- Bias due to deviations from intended interventions: This domain evaluates if participants are aware of their assigned intervention during the trial and if investigators are aware of participants' assigned intervention (study blinding).
- Bias due to missing outcome data: This domain evaluates if data for this outcome were available for all, or nearly all, participants who were randomized.
- Bias in measurement of the outcome: This domain evaluates the appropriateness of the method of measuring the outcome in the study and between the groups.
- Bias in selection of the reported result: This domain evaluates if the trial was analyzed in accordance with a pre-specified plan and there is no evidence of selection of the results.
- Overall risk of bias: This domain contains a summary of the risk of bias given by the review's authors (at least two different) on the base of the risk assessed in the previous five domains.

The risk of bias should also be graphically depicted with the dedicated Cochrane tool (Fig. 9.2).

For non-randomized studies other qualitative scales have been developed to assess the potential risk of bias. For surgical non-randomized studies one of the proposed scales is the MINORS (Methodological Index for NOn-Randomized Studies) which evaluates 12 items assessing all domains and possible source of biases [4].

Among all the possible biases the publication bias can be graphically depicted and evaluated with a specific graph: the funnel plot. The funnel plot is a scatter plot in which each dot represents a study, and it is allocated in the plot based on the study results (effect size on x axis) and the study precision (the inverse standard error or the number of cases, on y axis). If there is no publication bias the graph will represent an inverse funnel; in case a publication bias is present, the distribution of the dots will be skewed and asymmetric (Fig. 9.3).

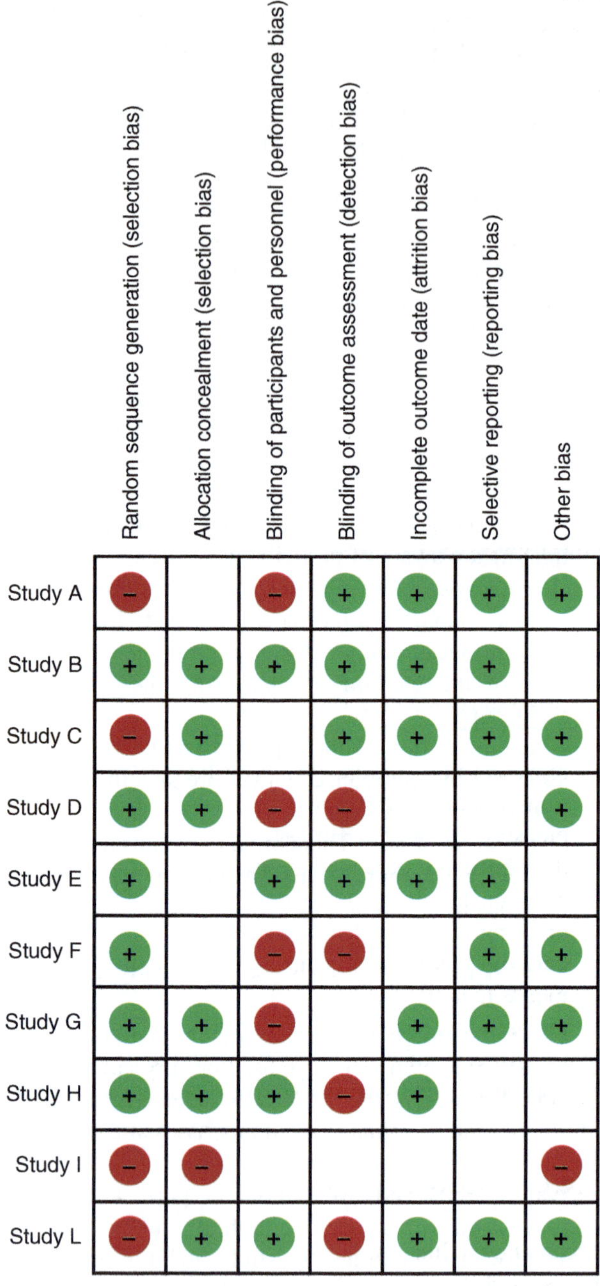

Fig. 9.2 Summary of risk of bias. The red dots indicate high risk of bias, green dots indicate low risk of bias, and white spaces indicated uncertain risk of bias

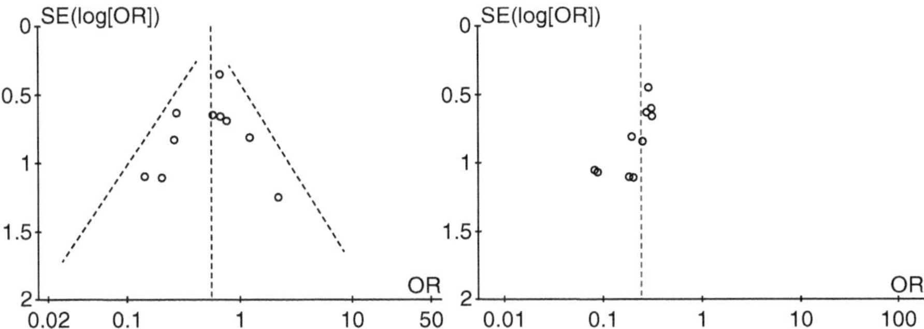

Fig. 9.3 Two example of funnel plots: on the left the distribution of studies is symmetrical (no publication bias); on the right the distribution of the studies is skewed (possible publication bias)

9.6 Results: Effect Measure

The main result of a meta-analysis is expressed with the effect measure. The effect measure is a statistical construct that compares outcome data between two intervention groups (intervention vs. control). The effect measure depends mostly on the type of data analyzed. Two general groups of effect measures exist: the ratio measures (for dichotomous outcomes) and the difference measures (for continuous outcomes).

According to the type of the data these are the most commonly adopted effect measures.

9.6.1 Binary Outcomes/Dichotomous Data

- Risk ratio (RR): It is the ratio between the risk of an event in the two different groups X and Y (see Chap. 8); it can be a number between 0 and infinite where 1 is the no effect value (same risk in the two different groups). When the risk of the event complication is higher in the laparoscopic appendectomy group than open appendectomy group, the RR will have value >1; on the contrary when the risk of the event is higher open appendectomy group than laparoscopic appendectomy group, the OR will have a value between 0 and 0.99. This is the preferred measure for randomized studies' outcomes. A RR = 1.56 should be interpreted as 56% higher risk of complications in laparoscopic appendectomy group compared with open appendectomy; RR = 0.56 should be interpreted as a 44% reduction of complication in laparoscopic appendectomy group.
- Odds ratio (OR): Similarly, to the RR this measure is the ratio between the odds of the event in the two compared groups (see Chap. 8). The measure is a number between 0 and infinity, where the value 1 corresponds to no effect (same odds in the two groups). When the probability of complication is higher in the laparoscopic appendectomy group than open appendectomy group, the

OR will have value >1; on the contrary when the probability of the event is higher in open appendectomy group, the OR will have a value between 0 and 0.99. Odds ratio should be adopted in meta-analysis of case–control studies. Differently from RR an OR = 1.56 does not correspond to a 56% increase in the risk! Its value could approximate the RR only when the frequency of the event is less than 10%.

9.6.2 Continuous Data (Also Scale Data or Counts of Events)

- Mean difference (MD): It measures the absolute difference between the mean values of two compared group, giving a numeric value that represents the pooled difference. The effect size provides information expressed as a clinical unit (for example, the mean difference of operating time, in minutes; Fig. 9.5). It is appropriate when all study results are expressed in the same measurement's unit.
- Standardized mean difference (SMD): When study results are available in different measurement units, continuous results can be meta-analyzed through the standardized mean difference that provides information expressed as statistical units. The standardized mean difference measures the effect on the base of data dispersion and it represents the effect expressed in number of standard deviations (SD) (differently from mean difference that is expressed in clinical unit as minutes, days, or milliliters of blood loss). A SMD of 1.1 represents a variation of 1.1 SD. Generally, the value 0.2 is considered as a small effect, 0.5 as medium, and 0.8 as large effect. This measure is not easy to be interpreted and it is useful in limited cases of surgical studies.

9.7 Results: The Forest Plot

Forest plots are the preferred graphs for reporting the results of meta-analysis. They contain several information about the meta-analysis. In this section we will show the forest plot created by the Cochrane RevMan software, the open-source tool provided by the Cochrane organization for making meta-analysis. Figure 9.4 shows the forest plot containing the results of our hypothetical meta-analysis with the comparison of a dichotomous outcome, morbidity rate, between laparoscopic and open appendectomy.

The forest plot is built as a combination of a table and a graph. On the left side are shown the results of each included study: the first line shows data about "Study A" with the number of events in the experimental and control treatment groups and the respective number of patients in each group. Each study has a "relative" weight in the meta-analysis: this weight is based on the study precision: the narrower is the 95% confidence interval (more precise data, small variance), the higher will be the weight; on the contrary, a study with a wide 95% confidence interval (CI) will have a lower weight. Finally, for each study is represented the effect estimate (the result of the study is represented with the chosen effect measure, along with its 95% CI).

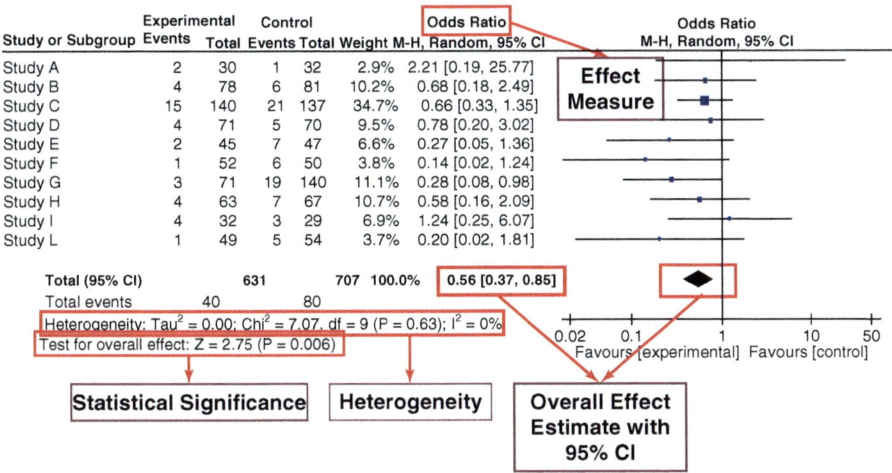

Study or Subgroup	Experimental Events	Experimental Total	Control Events	Control Total	Weight	Odds Ratio M-H, Random, 95% CI
Study A	2	30	1	32	2.9%	2.21 [0.19, 25.77]
Study B	4	78	6	81	10.2%	0.68 [0.18, 2.49]
Study C	15	140	21	137	34.7%	0.66 [0.33, 1.35]
Study D	4	71	5	70	9.5%	0.78 [0.20, 3.02]
Study E	2	45	7	47	6.6%	0.27 [0.05, 1.36]
Study F	1	52	6	50	3.8%	0.14 [0.02, 1.24]
Study G	3	71	19	140	11.1%	0.28 [0.08, 0.98]
Study H	4	63	7	67	10.7%	0.58 [0.16, 2.09]
Study I	4	32	3	29	6.9%	1.24 [0.25, 6.07]
Study L	1	49	5	54	3.7%	0.20 [0.02, 1.81]
Total (95% CI)		**631**		**707**	**100.0%**	**0.56 [0.37, 0.85]**
Total events	40		80			

Heterogeneity: Tau² = 0.00; Chi² = 7.07, df = 9 (P = 0.63); I² = 0%
Test for overall effect: Z = 2.75 (P = 0.006)

Fig. 9.4 A forest plot showing a comparison of a dichotomous outcome (complications following experimental treatment compared with control)

Study or Subgroup	Experimental Mean	Experimental SD	Experimental Total	Control Mean	Control SD	Control Total	Weight	Mean Difference IV, Random, 95% CI
Study A	120	18	30	118	35	32	4.7%	2.00 [−11.73, 15.73]
Study B	131	17	78	140	19	81	12.9%	−9.00 [−14.60, −3.40]
Study C	121	27	140	130	28	137	11.5%	−9.00 [−15.48, −2.52]
Study D	121	7	71	131	9	70	17.5%	−10.00 [−12.66, −7.34]
Study E	115	27	45	121	24	47	6.9%	−6.00 [−16.46, 4.46]
Study F	124	37	52	137	28	50	5.3%	−13.00 [−25.70, −0.30]
Study G	119	27	71	120	31	140	9.3%	−1.00 [−9.11, 7.11]
Study H	117	31	63	121	30	67	6.9%	−4.00 [−14.50, 6.50]
Study I	124	9	42	121	14	29	12.6%	3.00 [−2.78, 8.78]
Study L	131	16	49	137	15	54	12.2%	−6.00 [−12.01, 0.01]
Total (95% CI)			**641**			**707**	**100.0%**	**−5.69 [−9.12, −2.26]**

Heterogeneity: Tau² = 15.64; Chi² = 22.24, df = 9 (P = 0.008); I² = 60%
Test for overall effect: Z = 3.25 (P = 0.001)

Mean Difference IV, Random, 95% CI
−20 −10 0 10 20
Favours [experimental] Favours [control]

Fig. 9.5 A forest plot showing a comparison of a continuous outcome (operative time in minutes between two groups)

The effect measure is also depicted in the right part of the plot: the effect estimate is shown as a box and its dimension varies according to the study's weight (higher weight has bigger dimensions); the line represents the 95% CI.

The last line of the forest plot shows the results of the meta-analysis: the overall number of events and patients in experimental and control groups and the overall effect estimate. The effect estimate is a pooled estimation of the effect of all included studies, adjusted according to each study's weight. On the right it is shown as a diamond, having a width which represents the 95% CI.

On the right side, where effects are graphically shown, there is a vertical line: this line represents the line of "no effect." This line corresponds to the value "1" when the effect measure is a ratio (odd ratio, risk ratio) and the value "0" when the effect measure is a difference (risk difference, mean difference, standardized mean difference, see Fig. 9.5). The position of the diamond gives a graphical representation of the meta-analysis results: when the diamond lies entirely to one side of the line, there is a significant difference between the groups (the "no effect" value is not contained in the 95% CI). If the diamond is on the left of the line, the effect measure shows a lower frequency of events in the experimental group (a result favoring the experimental group in case of bad outcome, as complications or deaths, or favoring control group in case of good outcomes as cure, success of the therapy). On the contrary, if the diamond lies in the right of the line the result should be interpreted as favoring control group in case of bad outcomes.

On the bottom line there are information about the statistical heterogeneity (I^2) and the statistical significance of the analysis (test of overall effect Z).

In our hypothetical example, in which we analyzed the effect of laparoscopic appendectomy (experimental) compared with open appendectomy (control) on the complications rate, we included all the ten studies retrieved (from A to L). The overall effect showed a significant reduction of complications with laparoscopic appendectomy with an effect measure expressed as odds ratio of 0.56. This means that laparoscopic appendectomy reduced the complications by approximately 44% compared with open appendectomy. The confidence interval for the point estimates was 0.87–0.85.

Figure 9.5 shows the comparison of a continuous outcome (operative time) between our two chosen surgical interventions. The mean and the standard deviation for experimental and control groups are represented for each study; the weight of each study is calculated based on the data dispersion: higher SD corresponds to a lower weight. The chosen effect measure was the mean difference. The meta-analysis resulted in a significant reduction of operative time of −5.69 min (95% confidence interval −9.12; −2.26). We must notice that, despite statistical significance, the difference between the two treatments is clinically irrelevant (only 5 min difference).

9.8 Results: Heterogeneity

Heterogeneity is a fundamental aspect to be aware of when reading and performing a meta-analysis. It is defined as the presence of differences among studies. There are several kinds of heterogeneity:

- Clinical heterogeneity: A difference in the clinical setting or intervention of the included studies. This should be carefully described. If there was serious heterogeneity, then the meta-analysis may not be appropriate. An example, performing the same interventions (open versus laparoscopic appendectomy) but in different patients' populations (adult patients versus pediatric patients).
- Methodological heterogeneity: A difference in the study design. When present, the meta-analysis could be inappropriate. However, occasionally methodological heterogeneity can be overcome by using the subgroup analysis. An example for that is the presence of randomized and non-randomized studies in the same meta-analysis.

- Statistical heterogeneity: This indicates a difference in the results of the included studies. This may occur because the confidence intervals are not overlapping or because of differences in the direction and the magnitude of the effect of different studies. Statistical heterogeneity of the direction of the effect indicates that the beneficial or harmful effect of the treatment is not similar across the included studies. For example, in Fig. 9.4, in studies A and I the experimental treatment resulted in a harmful effect while in all the other studies had a beneficial effect: this represents a statistical heterogeneity.

Statistical heterogeneity is evaluated using the Chi squared test for heterogeneity with its *p*-value, indicated in the bottom line of the forest plot. A further evaluation is the inconsistency (the measure of incoherence among results), indicated by the I^2. I^2 represents the variation across studies due to heterogeneity. Generally, an I^2 value of less than 40% can be considered as not important, 40–75% as moderate, while more than 75% as substantial.

Heterogeneity conditions the calculation of the meta-analysis results. There are two statistical models for the calculation of the overall estimated effect: the fixed model and the random model. The fixed model is more accurate (narrower CI) but requires an absence of heterogeneity; the random model takes into account statistical heterogeneity and gives more solid results which avoid misinterpretations.

9.9 Interpretation of the Results

A meta-analysis is the result of a very complex and tedious work. The forest plot, that contains all the essential results, should be considered as "the tip of the iceberg" and the interpretation of the results should be a very accurate and cautious. When reading a meta-analysis, we must be familiar with the concept of certainty of the results, defined as the confidence that the true effect is within a particular range or threshold. In other words, certainty is the confidence that the pooled result is true and does not depend on heterogeneity and bias.

The point estimate of the measured effect gives us the direction and the magnitude of the effect. In Fig. 9.4 for example, the experimental treatment leads to a reduction of the outcome (complications) with a measured effect expressed as odd ratio of 0.56. This measure does not alone give us all the information we need to know. One of the most important information is the width of the confidence interval, in which we are 95% confident that the measured effect lies. In our example the confidence interval is between 0.37 and 0.85 giving us a reasonable certainty.

Great attention should be directed towards the difference between clinical and statistical significance: often, a statistically significant result (with a 95% confidence interval that does not contain the "no effect" value or a *p*-value <0.05) is not clinically significant. Figure 9.5 shows that the experimental treatment resulted in a lower operative time with a mean difference of −5.69 min (95% CI −9.12; −2.26). Although statistically significant, 5 min mean difference is clinically not important. Being expert in the studied area is very important to differentiate between clinical and statistical findings. We should not simply look through the narrow hole of the *p*-value.

The interpretation of the results when there is no significant difference between the two groups raises more difficulties. The absence of significant difference does not allow us to automatically conclude that the two compared treatments are equivalent. In this case, it is very important to differentiate between "true" no effect and uncertainty of the results, based on the evaluation of the width of the CIs.

9.10 Sensitivity Analysis

Since a meta-analysis is mainly a systematic review of the literature, there are several decisions that the researcher must take. Some of these decisions could be arbitrary and not objective. For example, the decision to adopt a numerical value as a cut-off for age, the decision to consider patients who were lost at follow-up as dead, or the decision to include or exclude a study for different reasons. All these elements could influence the results of the meta-analysis. Therefore, they should be analyzed with a sensitivity analysis, to evaluate their role as a possible source of variability. Sensitivity analysis is defined as a repetition of the analysis by changing the included elements or changing the arbitrary or unclear decision criteria. Sensitivity analysis evaluates the robustness of the results of the meta-analysis. The main factors that may implicate a sensitivity analysis are:

- the inclusion and exclusion criteria,
- the clinical or methodological design of studies (source of heterogeneity),
- the model adopted for the analysis,
- the effect measure chosen (for example, fixed effect vs. random effect, odd ratio vs. risk ratio).

Another example of a sensitivity analysis is the repetition of the analysis excluding studies by dimension (generally the exclusion of small studies) or by the presence of heterogeneity.

9.11 Common Mistakes Encountered in Submitted Systematic Review Manuscripts

These are some of the common mistakes we have encountered as reviewers in systematic review articles submitted to surgical journals that may lead to rejection of these papers. Highlighting these errors may help young researchers to avoid them. These errors include:

1. *Mixing between a systematic review, scooping review, and a narrative review*: A narrative review, although searches the literature, has a broad scope and does not follow the strict rules of systematic reviews which have a precise protocol

and search methods. It is subjective, affected by personal opinion and selection bias [5]. A scoping review, similar to systematic review should have a clear methodological protocol to reproduce the results [6]. It differs from a systematic review in two aspects: (1) including a minimum of one search engine, (2) having a broad research question [7], otherwise the methodology is the same.

2. *Unclear or unimportant research question*: It is very important to define an important focused research question. Systematic reviews may take up to 18–24 months of continuous work to be properly performed. Systematic reviews answering the same question will usually give the same answer if they follow the same methodology. Accordingly, it is important to check whether there are similar systematic reviews in the literature that answered the same question so this major effort can be utilized in the proper direction.
3. *Lack of a clear structured protocol*: This protocol should be written to be detailed so as to be followed when performing the study. It should define the search strategy, terms, outcome variables, and methods of statistical analysis.
4. *Lack of search experience*: Systematic reviews depend entirely on the search process. The literature search needs both a subject expert and a search methodologist to be useful. It should have enough technical details that can reproduce the study if done by others. This includes using appropriate truncations like (*) and using synonyms to assure retrieving and covering all core keyword variations and locating all possible evidence. For example, putting words between brackets will only search the exact sequence of the words and spaces and not individual words.
5. *Not properly following the protocol and inclusion exclusion criteria*: Systematic reviews by definition are original articles that have detailed methodology that can be reproduced by any researcher if methods were followed. The subjects of the study are the included articles. The authors should follow exactly the protocol of the study.
6. *Not documenting the search procedure*: This is a common mistake. The authors may really do a systematic review in a specific time using specific search engines and specific terms but do not document them. If not fully documented, the authors will not be able to reproduce the results. It is very important to document each step when doing the search so the PRISMA graph can be accurate and reproducible.
7. *Being too narrow in the search*: Some authors narrow the search without a justification to reduce the effort needed in performing a systematic review. They may narrow the period of the studies, the geographical location, or the search engines. A systematic review needs a minimum of two databases (we recommend at least PUBMED and EMBASE). The more databases are searched, the better the systematic review will be.
8. *Lack of critical appraisal and improper evaluation of the quality of the selected papers:* The authors should evaluate the quality of the studies even if the studies were retrospective. It is advised to have a minimum of two research methodologists who independently critically appraise the selected papers. This is very important to exclude papers being published twice either by increasing sample

size (in which the first should be excluded) or finding dual publication of the same data.

9. *Overusing statistics:* It is very important to know when not to do a meta-analysis. Just to clarify this issue, you cannot mix apples and oranges and count them together. Furthermore, adding combing weak studies or heterogenous studies does not increase the quality of the evidence.
10. *Not acknowledging biases*: The authors should recognize all relevant biases of a study including geographical bias, language bias, search bias, etc. This indicates that the authors were aware of the limitations of their study. It is advised to include this in detail in the limitations section [8].

9.12 Conclusions

Meta-analysis is a statistical technique that allows to combine the results of two or more studies. Meta-analysis cannot exist without a systematic review of the literature. Reading and understanding a meta-analysis is much more complex than looking at the forest plot. A "check-list" for a correct reading and interpretation of these complex studies includes:

- Accurate and precise literature review.
- Precise definition of inclusion and exclusion criteria.
- Description of retrieved studies with reasons for inclusion and/or exclusion.
- Assessment of the study quality and the potential risk of bias.
- Description of heterogeneity (clinical, methodological, and statistical).
- Evaluation of the correct effect measure.
- Assessment of statistical significance vs. clinical significance.

One of the commonest errors for the reader is to concentrate and give attention only to the forest plot drawing conclusions without critically reading the whole study. The robustness of the results should be accurately evaluated (with sensitivity analysis, for example). Even in case of statistically significant results (the diamond in the forest plot does not cross the no effect line), the presence of important heterogeneity could question the certainty of the results, and no definite conclusion can be reached. More specific and detailed description of the meta-analysis methodology can be found in the Cochrane handbook for systematic reviews and meta-analysis [1].

References

1. Higgins JPT, Thomas J, Chandler J, Cumpston M, Li T, Page MJ, et al. Cochrane handbook for systematic reviews of interventions. Oxford: The Cochrane Collboration and Wiley; 2019. https://training.cochrane.org/handbook. Accessed 2 Apr 2022.
2. Guyatt GH, Oxman AD, Vist GE, Kunz R, Falck-Ytter Y, Alonso-Coello P, et al. GRADE: an emerging consensus on rating quality of evidence and strength of recommendations.

BMJ. 2008;336:924–6. http://www.pubmedcentral.nih.gov/articlerender.fcgi?artid=2335261&tool=pmcentrez&rendertype=abstract.
3. Page MJ, McKenzie JE, Bossuyt PM, Boutron I, Hoffmann TC, Mulrow CD, et al. The PRISMA 2020 statement: an updated guideline for reporting systematic reviews. BMJ. 2021;372:n71.
4. Slim K, Nini E, Forestier D, Kwiatkowski F, Panis Y, Chipponi J. Methodological index for non-randomized studies (minors): development and validation of a new instrument. ANZ J Surg. 2003;73:712–6. http://www.ncbi.nlm.nih.gov/pubmed/12956787.
5. Papakostidis C, Giannoudis PV. Systematic reviews and meta-analyses: what are the common pitfalls? Injury. 2022;53:1301–4.
6. Tricco AC, Lillie E, Zarin W, O'Brien KK, Colquhoun H, Levac D, et al. PRISMA Extension for Scoping Reviews (PRISMA-ScR): checklist and explanation. Ann Intern Med. 2018;169(7):467–73.
7. Powell JT, Koelemay MJW. Systematic reviews of the literature are not always either useful or the best way to add to science. EJVES Vasc Forum. 2021;54:2–6.
8. Mohammad A, Branicki F, Abu-Zidan FM. Educational and clinical impact of Advanced Trauma Life Support (ATLS) courses: a systematic review. World J Surg. 2014;38:322–9.

10 Randomized Trials and Case–Control Matching Techniques

Emanuele Russo, Annalaura Montalti,
Domenico Pietro Santonastaso, and Giuliano Bolondi

10.1 Introduction to Randomized Trials

This chapter is intended as a general introduction on RCTs, discussing aims, strengths, and limitations, helping neophytes to interpret their results, without providing technical skills to perform them. In this section we will also address some issues related to case–control studies as they allow us to answer some questions that RCTs cannot answer.

Randomized control trials (RCTs) are considered one of the best and most rigorous clinical study designs available. They play a crucial role in expanding current medical knowledge, in reducing biases while experimenting a new treatment or approach and evaluating effectiveness and safety.

The history of RCTs is long: some rudimentary fundamentals are even found in the Bible: Two groups of youth were assigned to two different dietary regimens: the same foods as the King of Babylonia Nebuchadnezzar with a wine ration to one group and a teetotal vegan regimen to the other. The outcome was measured by the look of the faces at the end of the 10 days. By the way, vegans turn out to have a more florid appearance [1].

Initial attempts of structured clinical experiments have been conducted since the beginning of the eighteenth century about scurvy and then, more rigorously, during the first half of the twentieth century about tuberculosis [2–4].

E. Russo (✉) · D. P. Santonastaso · G. Bolondi
Anesthesia and Intensive Care Unit, AUSL Romagna,
Maurizio Bufalini Hospital, Cesena FC, Italy
e-mail: emanuele.russo@auslromagna.it; domenicopietro.santonastaso@auslromagna.it;
giuliano.bolondi@auslromagna.it

A. Montalti
Risk and Compliance, Healthcare, KPMG Advisory S.p.A., Milan, Italy

M. Ceresoli et al. (eds.), *Statistics and Research Methods for Acute Care and General Surgeons*, Hot Topics in Acute Care Surgery and Trauma,
https://doi.org/10.1007/978-3-031-13818-8_10

In RCTs, individuals are randomly assigned to either the experimental or the control groups. Treatment allocation should be blinded during the study and its data analysis (allocation concealment) when feasible. The object of the study can be clinical maneuvers, administration of drugs, diagnostic tests, surgery, protocol implementations, etc. [4].

In some cases, there are even more than two groups, for example, when testing different dosages of the same drug.

The enrolled subjects differ, by nature, for a large number of known and unknown characteristics, and not just for the experimental variable of interest: this complexity makes a crucial difference with lab-based experiments and the following data analysis. If the sample size is large enough, the randomization process ensures that these known and unknown variables are randomly distributed between the different experimental groups, not influencing the final result. The trial design itself and the data analysis techniques developed allow to recognize the presence of unmonitored differences between the groups.

Since 2004, a statement from the International Committee of Medical Journal Editors requires authors to register their studies and trials in public databases, certifying the respect of clear ethical and study design requirements (i.e.: www.clinicaltrials.gov) [5].

RCTs examine the effects of one or more contemporary interventions. The outcome variables measured can be clinical (survival, disease recurrence, hospital length-of-stay, rate of complications, etc.) or surrogates (physiological data or laboratory tests). *Surrogate outcomes* do not always prove to be clinically relevant: their interpretation can be unlinked to clinical outcomes, leading to uncertain interpretation, limiting the relevance and applicability of some studies. Surrogate outcomes that turn out to be related with clinical outcomes are defined as intermediate outcomes.

The "rough" nature of RCTs, merging together extremely different and complex individuals and trying to detect the impact of just a few experimentally controlled variables, has frequently led to non-significant results. For this reason, advanced data analysis methodologies have been developed.

Post-hoc subgroup analysis focuses on specific subsets of patients taking part in the RCT (i.e.: younger, sicker, etc.) and then re-runs the data analysis trying to identify whether the intervention could be effective in those subgroups. A rigorous report of the process and the results should be presented. The frequent overuse of post-hoc analysis deviates from the original design of the RCT, generating numerous problems: lower methodological accuracy, sample size inadequacy up to the risk of falsely statistically significant results [6, 7]. Subgroup analyses interpretation and their clinical application should be extremely cautious.

RCTs are not appropriate for the validation of screening tests and for the study of rare outcomes (because of the need for huge sample sizes) or long-term effects (unmodified group characteristics and strict follow-up are difficult to guarantee over years) [4].

10.1.1 Ethical Concerns Are Also Related to RCTs

The *World Medical Association Declaration of Helsinki (WMADH)* sets the ethical principles for medical research involving human subjects.

RCTs must not deprive patients of the best available treatments for their conditions. A strict surveillance for possible adverse effects or futility of the treatments must be ensured [8]. Finally, but not less importantly, studies in the emergency setting or about unconscious patients cannot, by definition, collect patients' informed consent.

A patient should be enrolled in a randomized clinical trial only if there is substantial uncertainty about which treatment is best. The aim is always to shed light on the interests of the future patient population.

When ethical questions are not clearly settled from RCTs, observational studies (OS) can still play a role [9]. OS have some advantages over RCTs, in particular lower costs and, frequently, less ethical concerns (lacking a direct intervention of the researchers on the population). However, the highest rate of biases of these studies places their results at a lower level of scientific relevance [10].

10.1.2 Placebo Effect

Finally, emotions, expectations, *placebo effects,* and the setting where the trial is performed can be important confounders of the measured outcomes; they might conceal the strength and effectiveness of the intervention. As stated in the review of Feyes et al., half of the overall effects observed are attributable to contextual effects rather than the intervention. The importance of contextual effects alongside the treatment should be considered and analyzed by researchers: this allows a deeper understanding of the overall benefits to patients [11].

Artificial intelligence and big data have started transforming clinical trials. Machine learning algorithms can be trained to select participants and end-points in a data-driven fashion. The integration between data science and RCTs is opening the doors towards greater efficiency and statistical power, overcoming the described limits of RCT [12].

10.2 Hypothesis Testing and Sample Size Calculation

The scientific method establishes a "*hypothesis testing*" approach to set up observational and experimental studies: the hypothesis is declared in advance and should be simple and specific. There are two types of hypotheses: the *null hypothesis (H_0)* and the one- or two-tailed hypothesis.

The null hypothesis states that there is no association between the predictor (or treatment) and the outcome variables in the population: if it is correct, the statistical test could predict the occurrence of an event by chance. On the contrary, the finding of a statistical association indicates that the alternative hypothesis (H_1) is true. The one-tailed hypothesis defines the direction of the association between the predictor and the outcome variables in the study population. The two-tailed hypothesis simply states that an association exists.

Statistical analyses of experimental data are affected by type-I and type-II errors. *A type-I error* (alpha) occurs when the examiner erroneously rejects the null hypothesis; for instance, it is mistakenly inferred that a treatment has a positive effect on a disorder. *A type-II error (beta)* occurs when the examiner erroneously accepts the null hypothesis [13].

Sample size is the number of cases (patients) enrolled in a trial. It should be estimated beforehand by a process known as *sample size calculation.*

Sample size calculation is a crucial step for the planning and the success of a RCT. According to the CONSORT (consolidated standard of reporting trials), in clinical research it is fundamental to report and to justify how the sample size is calculated [14].

The standard approach is to compute the sample size using four parameters: type-I error, power, variability (population variance of a given outcome variable), and the smallest treatment effect of interest.

Frequently, by convention, type-I error is set at 5% and the power (1 − type-II error) is set at 80–90%. The expected variability of the control group is specified on the basis of published results. The smallest treatment effect of interest is based on the expectations of the intervention and estimates from preliminary studies and explorative trials.

Many reliable sample size calculators are available online nowadays.

Thus, if a researcher wished to initiate a trial on a new suture material, he or she would first study the literature and estimate the benefit over the standard material used with respect to a predetermined outcome; then calculate the sample size and if the study did not reach the calculated size, it would probably be inconclusive.

Big sample sizes are very sensitive in detecting even the smallest differences, but may dramatically increase the costs. Underpowered sample sizes may fail to describe the effectiveness of a treatment, thus wasting the efforts of a research project without detecting any result. The calculation of the sample size helps to make clinical studies sustainable and powerful.

The statistical analysis requires, among the first steps, the detection of any significant differences in the distribution of covariates between groups (treatment vs. control).

The tests performed depend on the characteristics and distribution of the variables.

Significant differences in the distribution of outcome-related covariates across groups would need to be considered when interpreting trial results.

The hypothetical efficacy of the proposed treatment is tested with multivariate analysis techniques in which all possible variables related to the outcome are taken into account. The traditional model adopted for dichotomous outcomes is the binary logistic regression. Kaplan–Mayer or Cox regression is used for time-dependent outcome variables.

10.3 Reporting the Trials

Due to their complexity, it is frequently challenging to clearly communicate, through short scientific articles, all the relevant information concerning the trial. An expert reader (together with editors and reviewers involved in the publication process) should be able to make judgments regarding the internal and external validity of the trial [14].

To help this process and to set clear international standards, the CONSORT statement is a reference that is periodically updated and is endorsed by over 600 biomedical journals and editorial organizations. It provides a 25-topic checklist of information to include in a randomized trial report [15].

In accordance with CONSORT, it is mandatory to report data on: scientific background and explanation of rationale, specific objectives or hypotheses, eligibility criteria for participants, setting and allocation, interventions, outcomes, sample size, randomization, blinding, statistical method, participants flow, results, ancillary analysis, harms, limitations, generalizability, funding, and registration.

10.4 Randomized Controlled Trials Designs and Techniques

1. RCTs can be designed to test the *superiority, noninferiority, or equivalence* of two different treatments. The different perspective of these RCTs has evident consequences in their clinical interpretation.

   The superiority, noninferiority, or equivalence RCTs are characterized by different methodological features and statistical analysis.

   In superiority trials, the goal is to demonstrate that one treatment is better than another; for example, that one antibiotic achieves more clinical responses than another in the clinical resolution of ventilator-associated pneumonia from a specific bacterium. Sample size should therefore be calculated to test for significant differences between the two groups.

   In noninferiority trials, the goal is to demonstrate that one treatment is not inferior to another, e.g., an antihypertensive is not inferior to previous-generation treatments; the new, non-inferior, treatment might be preferred because it requires a single administration or has fewer side effects, this strategy may have business implications.

   From a statistical point of view, it is easier to demonstrate noninferiority than superiority.

   Equivalence studies aim to demonstrate that differences in the effectiveness of two treatments are within a range known as a margin of equivalence [16].
2. *Multicenter clinical trials* are fundamental in testing medical treatments and protocols. Based on the work of different clinical units, they should not be affected by local practices and patients' enrollment is expected to be faster, allowing the collection of a larger number of cases. These characteristics increase the generalizability of the studies.

This multicentric approach also shows some pitfalls: inter-site outcome differences are crucial to detect unexpected factors that could be unevenly distributed across clinical sites [17].

In multicenter trials it is therefore essential to verify the possible influence of the "center effect." The remarks on the Crash-2 trial are an interesting example for those interested in learning more about the topic [18, 19].

3. *Blinding*: This widespread technique reduces the information available to investigators, diminishing the probability of direct interventions and data manipulation due to unconscious expectations about what the tested approach should cause [20].

   These biases could affect the trial in any phase by any participant. Five categories involved in the study can be individuated and should be blinded whenever feasible: participants, clinicians, data collectors, outcome adjudicators, and data analysts. Unblinded participants, knowing the treatment or protocol they undergo, may modify their behavior, adherence, perception, or may show some placebo effect, altering the measured outcome. Unblinded clinicians are likely to influence their attitudes towards patients and data collection. Data collectors, outcome adjudicators, and statisticians should also be blinded to prevent biases on the analysis of the trial. Scientific, economic, professional, and other interests frequently put a significant pressure on the mentioned professionals and it has been demonstrated how this could affect results' accuracy.

   It must be specified in the study design and the final scientific report which individuals were blinded, how blinding was performed and whether they tested the successfulness of this strategy. Sometimes blinding is not physically possible (i.e.: testing a surgical versus pharmacological treatment is not hidden to the patients and the healthcare workers): it is possible to incorporate other methodological precautions, such as standardizing the treatment of the groups, considering an expertise-based trial design, using objective outcomes or acknowledging this limitation [21]. Finally, the study can be blinded to only some of the categories involved (patients, physicians, statisticians, etc.).

   The generic definitions "blind," "double-blind," etc. are discouraged because there is no homogeneity in their meaning. Instead, the categories undergoing blinding must be explicitly mentioned.

4. Different randomization designs are possible.
   (a) The most straightforward scheme for allocating subjects is *simple randomization*, using a single sequence of random assignments. The primordial method for simple randomization, adopted by Amberson in 1931, was to flip a coin to allocate the participants into two groups (treatment and control). Obviously, RCT randomization systems have been computerized nowadays.

      The method is easy and cheap to perform in clinical research. However, it could result in unequal numbers of participants in each group (mostly when small sample sizes are sufficient) or in groups with uneven covariates that make any clinical comparison unreliable [22, 23]. Simple randomization could also result in chronological biases if, by chance, one treatment is predominantly assigned earlier and the other later in time. To avoid these issues, *block randomization* can be used [24].

(b) B*lock randomization* creates blocks of random sequences, each block of equal size. This method assures a balance over time in the randomization between different groups. The above strategy is interesting for researchers managing small samples: being the blocks small, it is possible for the researchers to check and keep the number of participants in each group similar all the time. The blocks are generally composed of a multiple of the number of groups (i.e., with two treatment groups, the blocks are composed of four, six, or eight participants).

Once all possible balanced combinations of assignments are determined, the blocks are randomly chosen to determine the subjects' assignment into the groups.

However, groups are rarely comparable in terms of certain covariates (for example, it may be possible to find a higher incidence of a certain disease into a group), confounding results, making data analysis more challenging and clinical interpretation less reliable. It is recommended to test all those covariates that are expected to influence the measured outcome [24].

(c) S*tratified randomization* is used to balance the characteristics (covariates) of subjects among groups. The researchers must identify the specific covariates potentially influencing the measured outcome (dependent variable). The method sets up different blocks balancing different combinations of these covariates; the subjects are first assigned to the blocks representing their characteristics and then randomly assigned to the treatment or control arm of the study.

Stratified randomization decreases the probability of type-I error and increases the validity of subgroup and internal analysis [24]. It is a manageable and powerful tool for small clinical trials, it becomes complex when many covariates must be controlled.

A major limitation is that stratified randomization easily works when all the subjects have been identified before block assignment. In clinical research, subjects are enrolled on a continuous basis: their clinical characteristics are unknown at early stages of the study and the application of this method becomes challenging [23].

(d) *Adaptive randomization*

Adaptive randomization is a strategy to continuously balance the distribution of covariates across groups based on the previously enrolled cases. The probability of a patient to be assigned to any arm of the study is continuously recalculated based on the characteristics of the patients previously enrolled.

This method best performs in trials with small sample sizes. It requires continuous check of groups' characteristics and constant determination of the assignment of new patients. There are also randomization systems based on prior outcomes, but they are affected by a chronological bias and this may limit their validity.

(e) *Expertise-based trials*

The expertise of the practitioner about the different procedures tested in a trial can cause biases; measured procedural successes or failures might depend on the operators' skills. For instance, it is not appropriate to compare a laparoscopic procedure and a laparotomic procedure if the surgeon does not have an adequate case history of laparoscopy.

Some RCTs are designed so that the operators are only involved in procedures in which they can guarantee a predefined standard of care. This approach is also commendable from an ethical point of view.

The coordination between the randomization of enrolled subjects and the operators available in that precise moment can be a major challenge; moreover, a continuous check and intervention to balance covariates across groups must be guaranteed.

5. Experimental design

RCTs are also classified according to experimental design.

Parallel groups, based on allocation in the control or treatment group. Each patient can only receive one of the two treatments tested, e.g., neurosurgery versus endovascular treatment for a cerebral aneurysm.

Crossover trials: Group A and group B receive different treatments for a prespecified time, then it is inverted between the groups.

Cluster trials: Randomization is carried out not by single patient but by groups of patients (e.g., geographic area, hospital, school).

The majority of RCTs are studies with two arms of parallel groups [24].

6. Interim analysis

Interim analyses are conducted during the course of a trial, usually by independent agencies. Interim analyses are a means of securing ethical rigor of the trial.

It may happen that an RCT is stopped early because ongoing results show a very clear superiority of one treatment over another or harmful effects of a therapy. In these cases, it would be unethical to continue the study.

Interim analysis sometimes allows the sample size to be recalculated if the study design requires it.

10.5 Strengths of Randomized Trials

To date, RCTs are considered to provide the highest evidences, defining clinical decisions and being acknowledged as evidence of level A in current guidelines and reviews of the literature.

Randomization reduces the risk of several types of biases, generates comparable groups in terms of covariates, reducing the occurrence of not taking into account possible confounders. The different types of randomizations described above allow uniform groups to be exposed to controlled treatments and protocols (or placebo and standard of care).

Strictly applying standardized procedures, RCTs should ensure a continuous control of every step of the study. Scientific and statistical rigor and adherence to the experimental design generate univocal outcomes of clear interpretation and the possibility of generalizing them to similar settings [25].

RCTs are reliable in determining the cause–effect relation between treatment and outcome and if the outcome is clinically useful. Overtaking the limits of observational studies, RCTs ensure a higher control of the covariates that may influence the overall outcome [26].

10.6 Limitation of Randomized Trials

RCTs cannot be freely applied to every medical field. Despite being a "gold standard" for current research designs, the application of their results to the general population should always be very careful.

The randomization might cause the risk of *contamination*, selecting specific subpopulations and influencing the final results and their applicability to the general populations.

RCTs show limited power and efficacy for the study of complex traits (excessively variable phenotypes) or rare diseases (insufficient recruitable population) [27].

RCTs are time- and resource-consuming: possible conflicts of interests should be taken into account, forcing positive results or economically advantageous treatments. The conflict of interest is a "set of conditions in which professional judgment concerning a primary interest tends to be unduly influenced by a secondary interest" [28]. The danger from financial pressures on investigators and institutions is well described in the scientific literature [29]. The majority of medical studies are financed by private institutions instead of public funds or non-profit organizations: Bhandari et al. found that industry-founded trials are more likely to be associated with statistically significant findings in medical trials [30].

Considering the long-term effects of some interventions, RCTs definitive results are frequently available after a considerable time-span, terribly increasing the costs. Long lasting studies might suffer the risk of contamination between the experimental and the control arms, which increases over time [31].

The techniques used to improve RCTs quality and safety may result in biases and unreliable results too. This has been discussed in detail in Sect. 10.4 and is just briefly reviewed here.

Imperfect blinding and behavioral issues: The expectation of the trial and the placebo effect can influence the behavior of the subjects, investigators, the data analysis, and the results claimed [11].

In *multicenter studies* it is fundamental to check site-specific final differences to exclude unexpected confounders due to local clinical practices not addressed by the study design influencing the final results [32].

The CRASH-2 study is an example of a multicenter RCT suspected to be marred by possible site-specific effect. Moreover, limitations of this study have been raised with regard to some topics discussed in this chapter [18, 19]. Those interested in the debates regarding RCT limits can learn more by reading the discussions regarding the MERINO trial and CRASH-2 study [18, 19, 33–35].

10.7 Case–Control Studies and Case–Control Matching Techniques

Case–control studies are a sub-type of observational studies which often use matching factors. These research methodologies do not belong to the category of randomized trials; however, we consider appropriate to report a brief mention of them because this study design, diametrically opposed to RCTs, allows to answer questions to which trials cannot provide solutions.

Case–control studies compare retrospectively individuals who experience a condition of interest (cases) versus individuals who do not experience the condition (controls) with respect to exposure to a potential "risk factor." Controls must be selected from the same population from which cases were drawn.

This epidemiological study approach enables estimates of the relative risk of developing a disease or condition when a risk factor is present [36].

Case–control studies are often cheaper in terms of financial, logistical, and human resources than RCTs.

Case–control studies are considered efficient means of studying rare diseases with a long-term latency period. The best-known and most explanatory examples of case–control studies are the ones that have demonstrated the association between tobacco smoking and lung cancer in 50s. Furthermore, case–control studies may come in handy to investigate specific rare effects of a drug.

In case–control studies, matching techniques are often employed. Matching of cases is usually performed to control the effects of known potential confounding variables [19]. In small studies, they allow optimization of statistical power. For each enrolled case, a person with the same characteristics (age, sex, etc.) deemed relevant to the study is recruited into the control group.

Matching by age is suitable when studying risk factors for cancer, as both time of exposure and age of onset are relevant.

Therefore, an epidemiologist who wanted to study whether alcohol abuse is a risk factor for the development of breast cancer could conduct a case–control study, matching patients of the two groups for demographic characteristics, and other risk factors, first of all, age.

However, matching cases and control complicates the study, increases its cost, and exposes it to pitfalls in assessing the weight of variables.

Matching techniques fall into two main categories:

- Individual matching: Every case is matched to a control on the base of determined variables (e.g., age, gender, smoking status, etc.); it is possible also a different ratio (1:2, 1:4 case–control) according to the power analysis. Each case pair has identical values on the matching factors.

- Frequency matching: Matching occurs on the basis of the frequency distribution of the chosen variables within the group of cases. In addition, frequency matching uses multivariate analyses to control confounding [37].

However, if the matching is small, frequency matching can be futile.

Nowadays, computer algorithms are used to provide for the coupling between cases and controls.

10.8 Propensity Score and Inverse Probability

Introduced in 1983, "the propensity score is the conditional probability of assignment to a particular treatment given a vector of observed covariates" [38].

The propensity score (PS) is a coefficient estimating the probability of a case/patient to receive a specific treatment based on selected pre-existing covariates/characteristics.

The PS allows to design and analyze an observational (non-randomized) study in order to simulate some characteristics of a randomized controlled trial.

The propensity score also enables to calculate the inverse probability of treatment weights (IPTW) for each patient with simple mathematical formulas: 1/PS for patients receiving treatment and 1/(1 − PS) for patients not receiving treatment [39, 40].

For example, an observational study designed to test the outcome of severe traumatic brain injury patients intubated in the prehospital setting, versus those not intubated, could use a propensity score (estimated probability of being intubated based on neurologic status) to balance the nonrandomness of treatment.

The PS and IPTW play a balancing score role in observational studies: covariate adjustment, stratification or subclassification, and matching in case–control studies.

For example, a study with propensity score matching case–control techniques was used to investigate the influence of oral anticoagulation on stroke outcomes. The propensity score was used to match cases between different groups on prophylactic therapy with oral anticoagulants prior to the stroke event [41].

However, the use of inverse probability has some limitations. IPTW estimator does not perform properly with small samples; it is not yet proven to outperform multivariate logistic regression. Finally, the spread of PS and IPTW techniques has been increasing rapidly in recent years, but the adopted methodology is not always rigorous [39–42].

References

1. Holy Bible Book of Daniel (1; 1–21).
2. Amberson JB, McMahon BT, Pinner M. A clinical trial of sanocrysin in pulmonary tuberculosis. Am Rev Tuberc. 1931;24:401–35.
3. Streptomycin treatment of pulmonary tuberculosis. Br Med J. 1948;2(4582):769–82.

4. Stolberg HO, Norman G, Trop I. Randomized controlled trials. Fundamentals of clinical research for radiologists. Am J Roentgenol. 2004;183:1539–44. https://doi.org/10.2214/ajr.183.6.01831539.
5. De Angelis C, Drazen JM, Frizelle FA, et al. Clinical trial registration: a statement from the International Committee of Medical Journal Editors. N Engl J Med. 2004;351(12):1250–1.
6. Pocock SJ, Assmann SE, Enos LE, Kasten LE. Subgroup analysis, covariate adjustment and baseline comparisons in clinical trial reporting: current practice and problems. Stat Med. 2002;21(19):2917–30. https://doi.org/10.1002/sim.1296.
7. Horton R. From star signs to trial guidelines. Lancet. 2000;355(9209):1033–4. https://doi.org/10.1016/S0140-6736(00)02031-6.
8. World Medical Association. World Medical Association Declaration of Helsinki: ethical principles for medical research involving human subjects. JAMA. 2013;310(20):2191–4. https://doi.org/10.1001/jama.2013.281053.
9. Hannan EL. Randomized clinical trials and observational studies: guidelines for assessing respective strengths and limitations. JACC Cardiovasc Interv. 2008;1(3):211–7. https://doi.org/10.1016/j.jcin.2008.01.008.
10. Benson K, Hartz AJ. A comparison of observational studies and randomized, controlled trials. N Engl J Med. 2000;342(25):1878–86. https://doi.org/10.1056/NEJM200006223422506.
11. Feys F, et al. Do randomized clinical trials with inadequate blinding report enhanced placebo effects for intervention groups and nocebo effects for placebo groups? Syst Rev. 2014;3:14.
12. Lee CS, Lee AY. How artificial intelligence can transform randomized controlled trials. Transl Vis Sci Technol. 2020;9(2):9. https://doi.org/10.1167/tvst.9.2.9.
13. Banerjee A, Chitnis UB, Jadhav SL, Bhawalkar JS, Chaudhury S. Hypothesis testing, type I and type II errors. Ind Psychiatry J. 2009;18(2):127–31. https://doi.org/10.4103/0972-6748.62274.
14. Moher D, Schulz KF, Altman DG, CONSORT GROUP (Consolidated Standards of Reporting Trials). The CONSORT statement: revised recommendations for improving the quality of reports of parallel-group randomized trials. Ann Intern Med. 2001;134(8):657–62. https://doi.org/10.7326/0003-4819-134-8-200104170-00011.
15. Begg C, Cho M, Eastwood S, Horton R, Moher D, Olkin I, et al. Improving the quality of reporting of randomized controlled trials. The CONSORT Statement. JAMA. 1996;276(8):637–9. https://doi.org/10.1001/jama.276.8.637.
16. Piaggio G, Elbourne DR, Altman DG, Pocock SJ, SJW E, CONSORT Group FT. Reporting of noninferiority and equivalence randomized trials: an extension of the CONSORT Statement. JAMA. 2006;295(10):1152–60. https://doi.org/10.1001/jama.295.10.1152.
17. Ioannidis JPA, Dixon DO, McIntosh M, Albert JM, Bozzette SA, Schnittman SN. Relationship between event rates and treatment effects in clinical site differences within multicenter trials: an example from primary Pneumocystis carinii Prophylaxi. Control Clin Trials. 1999;20:253–66.
18. CRASH-2 Collaborators, Roberts I, Shakur H, Afolabi A, Brohi K, Coats T, Dewan Y, Gando S, Guyatt G, Hunt BJ, Morales C, Perel P, Prieto-Merino D, Woolley T. The importance of early treatment with tranexamic acid in bleeding trauma patients: an exploratory analysis of the CRASH-2 randomised controlled trial. Lancet. 2011;377(9771):1096–101, 1101.e1–2. https://doi.org/10.1016/S0140-6736(11)60278-X.
19. Mitra B, Mazur S, Cameron PA, Bernard S, Burns B, Smith A, Rashford S, Fitzgerald M, Smith K, Gruen RL. Tranexamic acid for trauma: filling the GAP in evidence. Emerg Med Australas. 2014;26:194–7.
20. Hróbjartsson A, Boutron I. Blinding in randomized clinical trials: imposed impartiality. Clin Pharmacol Ther. 2011;90(5):732–6. https://doi.org/10.1038/clpt.2011.207.
21. Karanicolas PJ, Farrokhyar F, Bhandari M. Practical tips for surgical research: blinding: who, what, when, why, how? Can J Surg. 2010;53(5):345–8.
22. Kao LS, Tyson JE, Blakely ML, Lally KP. Clinical research methodology I: introduction to randomized trials. J Am Coll Surg. 2008;206(2):361–9.
23. Suresh KP. An overview of randomization techniques: an unbiased assessment of outcome in clinical research. J Hum Reprod Sci. 2011;4:8–11.

24. Hopewell S, Dutton S, Yu LM, Chan AW, Altman DG. The quality of reports of randomised trials in 2000 and 2006: comparative study of articles indexed in PubMed. BMJ. 2010;340:c723. https://doi.org/10.1136/bmj.c723.
25. Deaton A, Cartwright N. Understanding and misunderstanding randomized controlled trials. Soc Sci Med. 2018;210:2–21. https://doi.org/10.1016/j.socscimed.2017.12.005.
26. Sibbald B, Roland M. Why are randomized controlled trials important? BMJ. 1998;316:201.
27. Hein S, Weeland J. Introduction to the special issue. Randomized control trials (RCTs) in clinical and community settings: challenges, alternatives and supplementary designs. New Dir Child Adolesc Dev. 2019;2019(167):7–15. https://doi.org/10.1002/cad.20312.
28. Thompson D. Understanding financial conflicts of interest. N Engl J Med. 1993;329:573–6.
29. Bekelman JE, Li Y, Gross CP. Scope and impact of financial conflicts of interest in biomedical research: a systematic review. JAMA. 2003;289(4):454–65. https://doi.org/10.1001/jama.289.4.454.
30. Bhandari M, Busse JW, Jackowski D, Montori VM, Schünemann H, Sprague S, Mears D, Schemitsch EH, Heels-Ansdell D, Devereaux PJ. Association between industry funding and statistically significant pro-industry findings in medical and surgical randomized trials. CMAJ. 2004;170(4):477–80.
31. Sason-Fisher RW, Bonevski B, Green LW, D'Este C. Limitations of the randomized controlled trial in evaluation population-based Health intervention. Am J Prev Med. 2007;33(2):155–61.
32. Kraemer HC, Robinson TN. Are certain multicenter randomized clinical trial structures misleading clinical and policy decisions? Contemp Clin Trials. 2005;26(5):518–29. https://doi.org/10.1016/j.cct.2005.05.002.
33. Harris PNA, Tambyah PA, Lye DC, et al. MERINO Trial Investigators and the Australasian Society for Infectious Disease Clinical Research Network (ASID-CRN). Effect of Piperacillin-Tazobactam vs Meropenem on 30-day mortality for patients with E coli or Klebsiella pneumoniae bloodstream infection and ceftriaxone resistance: a randomized clinical trial. JAMA. 2018;320(10):984–94. [Erratum in: JAMA. 2019 Jun 18;321(23):2370]. https://doi.org/10.1001/jama.2018.12163.
34. Rodríguez-Baño J, Gutiérrez-Gutiérrez B, Kahlmeter G. Antibiotics for ceftriaxone-resistant gram-negative bacterial bloodstream infections. JAMA. 2019;321(6):612–3. https://doi.org/10.1001/jama.2018.19345.
35. Missing information on sample size. JAMA. 2019;321(23):2370. [Erratum for: JAMA. 2018;320(10):984–994]. https://doi.org/10.1001/jama.2019.6706.
36. Pearce N. Analysis of matched case-control studies. BMJ. 2016;352:i969. https://doi.org/10.1136/bmj.i969.
37. Wachoider S, Silverman DT, McLaughlin JK, Mandel JS. Selection of controls in case-control studies. Am J Epidemiol. 1992;135(9):1042–50.
38. Rosenbaum PR, Rubin DB. The central role of the propensity score in observational studies for causal effects. Biometrika. 1983;70(1):41–55.
39. Chesnaye NC, Stel VS, Tripepi G, Dekker FW, Fu EL, Zoccali C, Jager KJ. An introduction to inverse probability of treatment weighting in observational research. Clin Kidney J. 2021;15(1):14–20. https://doi.org/10.1093/ckj/sfab158.
40. Schulte PJ, Mascha EJ. Propensity score methods: theory and practice for anesthesia research. Anesth Analg. 2018;127(4):1074–84. https://doi.org/10.1213/ANE.0000000000002920.
41. Rodríguez-Pardo J, Plaza Herráiz A, Lobato-Pérez L, Ramírez-Torres M, De Lorenzo I, Alonso de Leciñana M, Díez-Tejedor E, Fuentes B. Influence of oral anticoagulation on stroke severity and outcomes: a propensity score matching case-control study. J Neurol Sci. 2020;410:116685. https://doi.org/10.1016/j.jns.2020.116685.
42. Austin PC, Stuart EA. Moving towards best practice when using inverse probability of treatment weighting (IPTW) using the propensity score to estimate causal treatment effects in observational studies. Stat Med. 2015;34(28):3661–79. https://doi.org/10.1002/sim.6607.

Difference-In-Difference Techniques and Causal Inference

11

Sue Fu, Katherine Arnow, Amber Trickey, and Lisa Marie Knowlton

Research questions in medicine often center around measuring the effects of new treatments or interventions. We seek to study causal inference, the process of determining why certain outcomes occur. Randomized control trials, or RCTs, have long been considered the gold standard study design to measure the effect of an intervention. In a RCT, the randomization of study participants to a non-intervention and an intervention group is intended to eliminate any potential selection biases. By randomizing participation, the two groups should be balanced with regards to baseline characteristics, and therefore we can assume any differences in the outcomes between the two groups is attributable to the intervention alone. However, there are many disadvantages to RCTs. In the field of medicine and particularly in surgery, RCTs are often not feasible, from a practical, financial, or ethical perspective. Moreover, RCT study groups are typically carefully selected to control for unforeseen confounders. For example, researchers may restrict inclusion based on certain comorbidities, age, or sex when enrolling participants in a RCT. Therefore, the findings of RCTs may be challenging to generalize to the broader population. To illustrate using an actual study, a randomized control trial on operative versus antibiotic therapy for patients with appendicitis strictly limited participation in the antibiotic group to certain laboratory values and imaging findings, lack of appendicolith or leukocytosis within certain limits [1]. Consequently, the researchers cannot draw any conclusions on antibiotic therapy for patients outside those somewhat narrow parameters.

When randomization is not available or possible, researchers in surgery and other medical disciplines frequently conduct investigations using observational study methods, also known as quasi-experimental designs. Quasi-experimental

S. Fu (✉) · K. Arnow · A. Trickey · L. M. Knowlton
S-SPIRE, Department of Surgery, Stanford University, Stanford, CA, USA
e-mail: sfu87@stanford.edu; karnow@stanford.edu; Atrickey@stanford.edu; drlmk@stanford.edu

M. Ceresoli et al. (eds.), *Statistics and Research Methods for Acute Care and General Surgeons*, Hot Topics in Acute Care Surgery and Trauma,
https://doi.org/10.1007/978-3-031-13818-8_11

designs are empirical interventional studies that do not use randomization to assign study groups, but rather other criteria such as exposure to treatment or disease diagnosis. Particularly in the era of big data and sophisticated analytical tools, observational studies can offer considerable statistical power and relative ease of study implementation compared to randomized control trials. Large datasets, some of which are publicly available and follow thousands or even millions of individuals over time, present a rich resource for researchers. However, a disadvantage of quasi-experimental study designs is that they are subject to concerns of internal validity, as eligibility based on certain patient characteristics may impair the ability to draw conclusions on the effect of the intervention. How can researchers be sure that the intervention caused the change in outcome, rather than the inherent difference in patient characteristics that was used to determine participation in the non-intervention or intervention groups? This chapter will describe a commonly used quasi-experimental study design, difference-in-difference or DiD, that aims to answer this question and we will briefly discuss other quasi-experimental designs such as regression discontinuity, instrument variables, and synthetic controls.

If researchers want to assess the impact of an intervention using already available data, they can compare a group of individuals that received the intervention to a group that did not. When using retrospective data, it is imperative to account for all possible differences that existed before the intervention between the intervention and non-intervention groups for the purposes of internal validity. Yet this feat is virtually impossible because we lack perfect foresight to collect all possible relevant variables before conducting an observational study. Thus, it can be difficult to parse differences in the outcome of interest due to the intervention rather than the fundamental differences between the intervention and non-intervention groups. For instance, individuals in the intervention group may be more healthy or more sick at baseline or have greater or worse access to healthcare compared to people in the non-intervention group. These factors can significantly affect the outcome of interest and therefore constrain researchers' ability to meaningfully draw any conclusions regarding the intervention in question.

As a practical example of selection bias, several retrospective cohort studies compared two treatments for aortic valve replacement. These studies compared the Ross procedure which utilized an autograft to versus mechanical valve replacement with optimal anticoagulation therapy and studied the outcome of overall survival. Overall the studies found that survival of patients undergoing the Ross procedure was better than those who underwent a mechanical valve replacement [2, 3]. However, these studies could not rule out bias due to patient selection, as patients who received the Ross procedure tended to be younger and in better physical condition. How could the researchers know that the improvement in survival of patients receiving the Ross procedure was attributable to the supposed superiority of the Ross procedure to mechanical valve replacement, rather than the patient's relative youth and physical fitness?

Fortunately, there are various statistical methods that can account and control for pre-intervention differences between study groups. One technique is the difference-in-difference method. DiD first originated in economics and is now frequently used across health and health-related specialties, particularly to measure the effect of a health policy change [4]. DiD compares the changes in outcomes over time between a cohort which experienced the intervention or exposure and a non-intervention cohort which did not receive the intervention or exposure. It is well suited to evaluating the outcomes of health policy changes because it allows researchers to account for secular changes, i.e. changes that would have occurred over time sans intervention and therefore isolate the causal effect of the intervention in question. DiD has been used to evaluate policies such as the 2011 Accreditation Council for Graduate Medical Education resident duty hour reforms in the United States [5], and the Affordable Care Act [6]. With resident duty hour reform, safety outcomes were compared in teaching hospitals (the intervention group) to non-teaching hospitals (the non-intervention group) before and after implementation of the 2011 reform. We will delve more deeply into this study as an example later in the chapter. As another example, the effect of the Affordable Care Act on access to rehabilitation centers for adults after traumatic injury has been studied by comparing outcomes in states that expanded Medicaid eligibility to states that did not expand Medicaid before and after expansion in 2014 [6].

Figure 11.1 illustrates the DiD approach with a simplified example. The outcome of interest before and after the intervention is compared between the non-intervention group which does not undergo the intervention (group N) and the intervention group which does experience the intervention (group I). The difference in outcomes for group I before and after the intervention is represented by I2 – I1, and the difference in outcomes for group N after the intervention is represented by N2 – N1. Therefore,

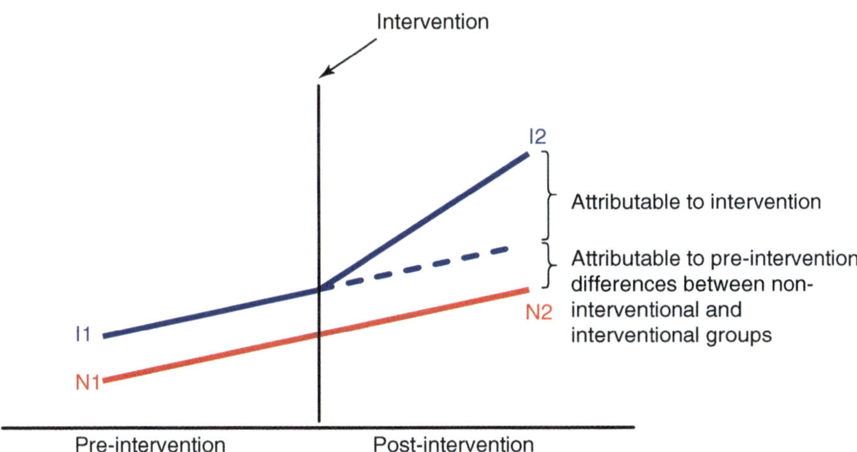

Fig. 11.1 Difference-in-differences graph

the change in outcome that is attributable to the intervention that is separate from the change in outcomes based on the inherent differences between groups N and I is the difference-in-difference estimate, which is equal to (I2 – I1) – (N2 – N1). The dotted line represents the outcomes for group I had been no intervention. If there had been no intervention, the difference-in-difference estimate would be equal to zero because the difference in group I over time is equal to the difference in group N over time.

Imagine that some hospital decided to use a new sterilizing technique, while hospital decided to use the old sterilizing method. The infection control committee is interested in measuring the rate of surgical site infections after this new sterilization technique was introduced. For a difference-in-difference study, the researchers measure the surgical site infection rate between the hospitals using the new sterilization technique and the hospitals using the old technique before and after the new sterilization technique was introduced. Figure 11.2 shows a table of the surgical site infection rates with this data.

In our simplified example, the difference-in-difference in surgical site infections attributable to the new sterilization technique is a decrease of 5%. Therefore the infection control committee can conclude that the new sterilization technique is associated with a 5% decrease in surgical infection rates.

In practice, regression models are used to produce the DiD estimates, rather than these simplified subtraction models. Most statistical software packages have difference-in-difference commands and programs. DiD studies can use linear or logistic regression models, or even more complex regression types. Linear regression is used when the outcome variable is continuous, such as financial costs or rates of mortality. Logistic regression is used when the outcome is dichotomous, such as presence or absence of a complication. In the regression model, the DiD estimate is the interaction term between time and the treatment groups. If the interaction term is significantly different from zero, then it can be concluded that there is an association between the intervention and the outcome of interest. The DiD results can be plotted graphically over time, comparing the outcomes between the two groups before and after the intervention. Results are also often reported in tables, with the actual difference-in-difference estimate, the interaction term between time and treatment groups in the regression model. In our made-up example of surgical site

	Before introduction of new sterilization technique	**After introduction of new sterilization technique**
Surgical site infections in hospitals using the new technique	6%	1%
Surgical site infections in hospitals using the old technique	3%	2%

Difference-in-difference = (1%–6%)–(2%–3%) = –5%

Fig. 11.2 Simplified example of DiD

infections after a new sterilization technique, there might be other factors the researchers want to adjust for, such as operation type, patient comorbidities, and surgical volume. They would need to perform a linear regression model to adjust for all these factors. The main dependent variables in the regression model would be time, marked as before and after the introduction of the new sterilization technique, as well as intervention vs. non-intervention hospitals, and the interaction between time and intervention groups. The regression would then adjust for other covariates, such as patient comorbidities, operation type, and surgical volume. Ultimately, the interaction term between the time variable and the sterilization technique groups is the final difference-in-difference estimate.

An actual example of difference-in-difference methodology in practice comes from a study from the United States on patient outcomes after the 2011 Accreditation Council for Graduate Medical Education (ACGME) resident duty hour reform by Rajaram et al. [5]. On July 1, 2011, the ACGME implemented additional resident duty restrictions training in the United States, including limiting first year trainees to 16 hours of continuous in-hospital clinical duty, 8 hours free between shifts, and residents on 24 hour shifts must have 4 hours for transfer of care activities with at least 14 hours off between shifts. The duty hour restrictions aimed to reduce preventable medical errors due to resident exhaustion. However, there were mixed opinions regarding the policy's potential efficacy. Opponents to the reforms believed that increased sign-outs and changeovers in care would possibly worsen patient outcomes, while proponents believed the duty reform hours would help reduce resident errors and improve patient safety.

To answer the question of whether patient outcomes were affected by the resident duty hour reforms, a study was undertaken to measure mortality and serious morbidity at 2 years prior and after the 2011 reforms [5]. Patient outcomes at teaching hospitals with residents were compared to non-teaching hospitals. Ultimately, over 200,000 patients from 23 teaching hospitals and 31 non-teaching hospitals were studied. The mortality and serious morbidity rate was 11.6% in teaching hospitals in 2009–2010 and 9.4% in 2012–2013, whereas it was 8.7% in 2009–2010 and 7.1% in 2012–2013 in non-teaching hospitals. After logistic regression, which adjusted for factors such as patient age, comorbidities, and illness severity, the odds ratio (OR) of death or serious morbidity was not statistically significant from 1 (OR 1.06, confidence interval 0.93–1.20) between teaching hospital and non-teaching hospitals. Recall that an odds ratio of 1 means that there is no difference in the likelihood of an outcome in the test group compared to the control group. Therefore, the study concluded that there was no associated change on patient safety and outcomes from resident duty hour reforms.

In the prior example of resident duty hour reforms, the intervention group were the patients who were treated at teaching hospitals. The non-intervention group were patients who were treated at non-teaching hospitals. The intervention under study was the 2011 resident duty hour reforms. The researchers showed their results in graphs depicting mortality and serious morbidity complication rates between teaching hospitals and non-teaching hospitals at 6-month intervals from January 2009 to July 2013. Graphs like these are helpful to visualize the overall trend in outcomes between the intervention and non-intervention groups. Additionally, the researchers in the Rajaram et al. study also looked at other patient outcomes, such as surgical site infections, sepsis or septic shock, as well as resident education outcomes such as test scores on the American Board of Surgery In-Training Examination. They then used tables to report their results of their difference-in-difference estimates of all the outcomes they studied.

There are certain criteria to conduct a DiD study. For one, longitudinal or panel data is required. Longitudinal data follows large groups of people over a long time. Panel data is a type of longitudinal data that contains observations of different cross-sections across time. For example, the 2011 resident duty reform study used panel data of patients who underwent surgery in 2009–2010 and 2012–2013. The key is that the same or equivalent cohorts are studied before and after an intervention. Additionally, DiD analysis relies on several assumptions. The main assumption is that the intervention and non-intervention groups must display parallel trends in outcome. This means that in the absence of any intervention, the difference between the intervention and non-intervention groups would be the same over time. This cannot be proven empirically, but statistical tests and visual validation of pre-intervention data can establish sufficient parallel trends. In the Rajaram et al. study, the graphs showing mortality and serious morbidity rates between the teaching and non-teaching hospitals stayed relatively parallel, confirming that there was no difference in patient outcomes associated with resident duty hour reform. Another assumption is called common shocks, which requires that any event that occurs during or after the intervention should equally affect both groups. The 2011 duty hours did not experience such a shock, but let us suppose that there was a world-wide pandemic during the time of the study which would have impacted teaching and non-teaching hospitals equally. In addition to these assumptions, other limitations of DiD include the necessity to account for spillover effects. Spillover occurs when the policy affects other aspects of clinical care which may influence the intervention or non-intervention group. For example, in the sterilization technique example, the sterilization technique might also affect food safety in the hospital, which could also affect nutritional status of patients and therefore patient outcomes.

There are additional statistical methods that can be used to further reduce confounding factors, such as propensity score matching, weighting, or stratification [7]. These techniques can be used in combination with DiD or other quasi-experimental designs. Other quasi-experimental methods that can be used to deduce causal inference when randomization is not available include regression discontinuity, instrumental variables, and synthetic controls. Regression discontinuity measures the effect of an intervention by assigning intervention and non-intervention groups based on a threshold cutoff of a continuous variable. An example of this exists in the United States with Medicare. Eligibility for Medicare, which is government sponsored health insurance occurs at 65 years of age; however, 64-year-old individuals are likely quite similar to 65-year-old individuals with the exception of their guarantee of health insurance coverage. This provides an opportunity to study how access to insurance may affect health outcomes by evaluating the difference between

64-year-old individuals and 65-year-old individuals. There was a study that used regression discontinuity to measure health outcomes after age 65 based on the hypothesis that nearly universal health coverage would be associated with positive changes in health outcomes. This study found that certain low-income minorities saw significant increases in self-reported health after age 65 [8].

Instrumental variables are another research tool to exploit naturally occurring phenomena to circumvent traditional randomized study design. The instrumental variable is a proxy for randomization of the explanatory variable but it itself cannot be related to the outcome. For example, geographic distance to hospitals or specialty centers is often used as an instrumental variable. Geographic distance affects access to timely and appropriate care but does not, by itself, affect health outcomes. In a study of mortality after traumatic injury, researchers used ambulance transport time to naturally randomize patients based on injury severity and other patient baseline characteristics [9]. Other commonly used instrumental variables in medicine include genotype, physician or institution preference expressed by patients, or prescribing trends over time.

Synthetic controls are yet another tool to estimate the effect of an intervention or treatment in the absence of randomization. With synthetic controls, the comparison cohort is constructed from a weighted combination of several non-intervention groups, and therefore useful when there is no natural comparison control group. An example is a study on pre- and post-bariatric surgery health utilization outcomes that used a synthetic control to compare health care utilization between individuals who had not undergone bariatric surgery to those who had [10]. The researchers used claims data to analyze health care costs of patients who underwent bariatric surgery, however their data set did not have a group of untreated patients that they could compare to, so they constructed a synthetic control using covariates that were related to healthcare costs. Overall they found bariatric surgery was associated with decreased costs in medication, especially for cardiovascular and diabetes treatment, as well as physician services. However this was offset by increased inpatient services after surgery.

In summary, randomized control trials remain the most robust study tool to measure causal inference, as the randomization process is the best to eliminate patient selection bias. However, they are often costly both in time and money and may not be ethically feasible. Quasi-experimental designs, such as difference-in-difference, have the advantage of being relatively intuitive and comparatively easier to implement than RCTs because researchers can use already available data. Difference-in-difference is a particular type of quasi-experimental study that can be used to assess the impact of a policy change, such as laws or public health policy or institutional reforms. However it requires a robust control group that is well defined and the data must meet the assumption that the intervention and non-intervention groups would have performed the same in the absence of the intervention. Other quasi-experimental designs exists, including regression discontinuity, instrumental variables, and synthetic controls. All these methods have their advantages and can be used in certain study scenarios. These techniques can also be limited by their strict criteria. Nonetheless, they are powerful tools for researchers for the right question.

References

1. CODA Collaborative, et al. A randomized trial comparing antibiotics with appendectomy for appendicitis. N Engl J Med. 2020;383:1907–19. https://doi.org/10.1056/NEJMoa2014320.
2. Andreas M, Wiedemann D, Seebacher G, Rath C, Aref T, Rosenhek R, et al. The Ross procedure offers excellent survival compared with mechanical aortic valve replacement in a real-world setting. Eur J Cardiothorac Surg. 2014;46:409–14. https://doi.org/10.1093/ejcts/ezt663.
3. David TE, David C, Woo A, Manlhiot C. The Ross procedure: outcomes at 20 years. J Thorac Cardiovasc Surg. 2014;147:85–94. https://doi.org/10.1016/j.jtcvs.2013.08.007.
4. Dimick JB, Ryan AM. Methods for evaluating changes in health care policy: the difference-in-difference approach. JAMA. 2014;312:2401. https://doi.org/10.1001/jama.2014.16153.
5. Rajaram R, Chung JW, Jones AT, Cohen ME, Dahlke AR, Ko CY, et al. Association of the 2011 ACGME resident duty hour reform with general surgery patient outcomes and with resident examination performance. JAMA. 2014;312:2374–84. https://doi.org/10.1001/jama.2014.15277.
6. Zogg CK, Scott JW, Metcalfe D, Gluck AR, Curfman GD, Davis KA, et al. Association of Medicaid expansion with access to rehabilitative care in adult trauma patients. JAMA Surg. 2019;154:402–11. https://doi.org/10.1001/jamasurg.2018.5177.
7. Stuart EA, Huskamp HA, Duckworth K, Simmons J, Song Z, Chernew M, et al. Using propensity scores in difference-in-difference models to estimate the effects of a policy change. Health Serv Outcomes Res Methodol. 2014;14:166–82. https://doi.org/10.1007/s10742-014-0123-z.
8. Card D, Dobkin C, Maestas N. The impact of nearly universal insurance coverage on health care utilization: evidence from Medicare. Am Econ Rev. 2008;98:2242–58. https://doi.org/10.1257/aer.98.5.2242.
9. Newgard CD, Schmicker RH, Hedges JR, Trickett JP, Davis DP, Bulger EM, et al. Emergency medical services intervals and survival in trauma: assessment of the "Golden Hour" in a North American Prospective Cohort. Ann Emerg Med. 2010;55:235–246.e4. https://doi.org/10.1016/j.annemergmed.2009.07.024.
10. Kurz CF, Rehm M, Holle R, Teuner C, Laxy M, Schwarzkopf L. The effect of bariatric surgery on health care costs: a synthetic control approach using Bayesian structural time series. Health Econ. 2019;28:1293–307. https://doi.org/10.1002/hec.3941.

Machine Learning Techniques

12

Jeff Choi, Nima Aghaeepour, and Martin Becker

12.1 Machine Learning and Artificial Intelligence

Machine learning comprises algorithms that can perform tasks they were not explicitly programmed to perform. Explicitly programmed algorithms perform tasks according to a predefined sequence of instructions. Conversely, machine learning algorithms are programmed to *learn to* perform tasks using input data. In the era of abundant data, affordable data storage, and computational capabilities, understanding machine learning algorithms is critical to better explore and answer questions that can advance surgical science.

This chapter will introduce machine learning terminology, common algorithms, and considerations for applying and fine-tuning algorithms. Our hope is that this overview will allow surgeons and surgeon scientists to better interpret machine learning algorithms in literature and understand which algorithms may be most appropriate to answer their research questions.

12.2 Machine Learning Terminologies and Concepts

12.2.1 Algorithms, Models, Inputs, and Outputs

Most machine learning algorithms aim to derive "**models**" from given data. This derivation process is called the "**training**" phase in which "the model is trained" and the data used to derive/train the model is called the "training data." The resulting models are then able to produce an estimated output (e.g. inpatient mortality) from inputs (e.g. demographic and hospitalization variables). In the statistical

J. Choi · N. Aghaeepour (✉) · M. Becker
Stanford University, Stanford, CA, USA
e-mail: jc2226@stanford.edu; naghaeep@stanford.edu; mgbckr@stanford.edu

M. Ceresoli et al. (eds.), *Statistics and Research Methods for Acute Care and General Surgeons*, Hot Topics in Acute Care Surgery and Trauma,
https://doi.org/10.1007/978-3-031-13818-8_12

learning framework of output = f (input), synonyms for inputs include "independent variables," "predictors," and "features," while synonyms for outputs include "dependent variables," "prediction," and "outcomes." Here f represents a model which is derived by applying a given machine learning algorithm to given training data. Models can solve different problem settings such as **classification** or **regression**. Classification involves predicting discrete outputs (e.g. surviving vs. not surviving hospitalization), while regression involves predicting a continuous output (e.g. hospital length-of-stay).

Each model has ***model parameters*** (also called *learnable parameters* or simply *parameters*) that are derived during the training phase. These model parameters specify how the model maps inputs to outputs. For example, in linear regression, these model parameters correspond to the model coefficients, and for deep learning models model parameters comprise weights (for more details, see Sect. 12.3). Often machine learning algorithms have parameters themselves which govern the way model parameters are derived from the data (e.g. such a parameter may trade off how quickly the training will finish vs. how accurate the model will be). Such parameters are called ***hyperparameters***.

Note that in practice, the term "**algorithms**" and "**models**" are sometimes used interchangeably.

12.2.2 Dimensions

Most researchers are familiar with clinical data in the tabular form of an $N \times M$ matrix, where N (number of rows) represents the number of subjects and M (number of columns) represents the number of different variables stored per patient. Each input variable constitutes a **dimension**. For example, if data comprises five variables for 50 patients, the input features encompass five dimensions. To reiterate, dimensionality refers to the number of input variables, *not* the number of subjects.

Overall, more *samples* are generally better for machine learning algorithms. However, while more input variables contain more information and may thus allow to build more powerful models, at the same time, the "curse of dimensionality" refers to potential issues that arise as the number of input variables grows and can make training machine learning models challenging and result in underperforming models. To handle large amounts of input variables, feature selection and dimensionality reduction are useful tools which we cover later in this chapter. First, for understanding the curse of dimensionality it is important to understand the concepts of overfitting vs. underfitting and bias vs. variance as outlined below.

12.2.3 Overfitting vs. Underfitting

When researchers build an algorithm, the hope is that the algorithm will be used by others in "the real world." **Overfitting** is a phenomenon when the algorithm has good results on the population it was built on, but has poor generalizability to other populations. For example, if a mortality-prediction algorithm accurately predicts mortality among patients whose data informed algorithm development (the training data), but has poor predictive capacity when used in other hospitals, the algorithm lacks generalizability and was overfit.

High-dimensionality (too many input variables) begets overfitting. Consider Dataset A, which recorded 5 variables for 100 subjects, and Dataset B, which recorded 50 variables for 100 subjects. Compared to Dataset A, Dataset B is much more likely to have unique rows (combination of values for 50 variables). And if each patient in Dataset B is uniquely identifiable, this would allow a model to learn output variables by sample rather than learning a more meaningful relationship between the input and output variables. Since the model is then based on identifying individual samples, it would not produce accurate predictions on unseen data. Thus it is not generalizable to other populations that may have different combinations of values for the same 50 variables.

However, for overfitting intrinsically powerful models are required. In contrast, if an algorithm is too simplistic to capture the underlying relationship of input and output variables, or has to work with too few variables as input that do not capture the output, the resulting model may suffer from underfitting. For example, linear models (like logistic regression) will never be able to capture non-linear relationships between input and output features, no matter how many subjects are in a dataset. Similarly, if the only input variable available is *sex*, no algorithm could accurately predict mortality.

Overfitting suffers from high variance, whereas **underfitting** suffers from high bias as introduced below. Selecting the optimal machine learning algorithm requires understanding the tradeoff between overfitting and underfitting and the tradeoff between bias and variance.

12.2.4 Bias vs. Variance Tradeoff

Understanding the bias and variance tradeoff first requires acknowledging that no algorithm is built using complete data. Complete data would encompass every member of a population of interest, and knowing all variables and variable value combinations for every member that could reasonably inform an output. Complete data is unobtainable, and all machine learning algorithms are built using incomplete data: a limited sample cohort from the population of interest and a limited number of variables from all variables that could inform an outcome.

Because algorithms are built using incomplete data, outputs are derived in the form, *output = f(input) + error*. "**Error**" determines how different the true output is from the calculated output. "Error" comprises variance, bias, and irreducible error. Irreducible error cannot be reduced by any algorithm and is a limitation of having incomplete data (e.g. unknown variables that actually affect how inputs map to outputs).

Variance explains how much a model's predictions vary given small data variations, e.g. in different data cohorts. For example, as mentioned previously, applying an algorithm of sufficient flexibility to too many input variables may result in overfitting, which manifests as high variance. **Bias**, however, explains how much the average prediction of an algorithm differs from the actual result. For example, an algorithm that is not flexible enough may not be able to learn the underlying relationship of inputs and outputs and thus is prone to underfitting, which manifests as high bias.

Why is there a tradeoff between bias and variance? As there are more input variables relative to the number of samples, variance will generally increase, and bias will decrease for a sufficiently flexible model. Conversely, when a model with less flexibility is applied, variance will generally decrease but bias will increase. Remember that a model's output error comprises variance, bias, and irreducible error. The former two are tightly connected to model flexibility, while the irreducible error is a consequence of data limitations such as missing important variables or not enough data. Training an optimal model requires selecting an algorithm of appropriate flexibility and selecting the number of input variables that will minimize the total error (minimum combined variance and bias) in the "real-world" population.

12.2.5 Model Flexibility

The bias and variance tradeoff also concerns different types of algorithms and their flexibilities. The third section of this chapter (Sect. 12.3) will explore common machine learning algorithms in depth, but we will briefly introduce the concept of **model flexibility**. There are many types of machine learning algorithms. Most readers are likely familiar with linear regression models and may have heard of deep neural networks. Linear regressions are much less flexible compared to deep neural networks. Without getting into complex mathematics, model flexibility can be conceptualized as the complexity of paths that map inputs to an output. For example, linear regression maps a simple, linear relationship from inputs to an output (little flexibility), whereas deep neural networks can map more complex relationships between inputs and the output.

As such, flexible models are more likely to accurately predict an output that matches the truth (low bias), but risk overfitting (high variance), particularly when a large number of variables is available. Simpler, less flexible models tend to have higher bias, but less variance. Thus, as discussed above, it is important to consider the bias–variance tradeoff when choosing the type of machine learning algorithm as well as its configuration, in addition to selecting the number of input variables.

12.2.6 Feature Selection and Dimension Reduction

With ubiquitous omics (e.g. radiomics, transcriptomics) technologies and electronic health records, modern medicine produces abundant variables to integrate into models. In combination with comparably small sample sizes, building optimal models often requires methodically decreasing the complexity of the data by reducing the number of input variables in order to prevent overfitting and allow for generalization. Reducing the number of variables can be done based on domain knowledge *before* analyzing the data or *integrated into the training phase*. Two specific strategies to narrow the list of inputs in the training phase are "feature selection" and "dimensionality reduction."

Feature selection involves *selecting* input variables that will likely inform the best model. For example, if the candidate input variables to predict mortality were (*age, co-morbidity A, co-morbidity B, disease A, disease B*), feature selection may lead to selecting (*age, co-morbidity A, disease B*) as the final input variables. Importantly, since feature selection requires considering the output of the model to evaluate its performance as features are selected, *feature selection must only be applied on the training set* explicitly excluding samples from the test set. A brute force approach to feature selection may entail fitting models with all possible combinations of candidate input variables (e.g. if there are 7 possible input variables, 2^7 models would be fit) and selecting the model with the best performance. Several performance metrics have been developed to penalize models with a higher number of variables and can help to choose optimal models. Examples of such metrics are Cp, Akaike information criterion (AIC), and adjusted R^2. In brief, lower Cp values, lower AIC, and higher adjusted R^2 indicate better models.

If a research question has many candidate input variables, feature selection can be complex and computationally expensive. There is a wide variety of computationally more efficient alternatives. For example, features can be selected based on univariate analysis of their relation to the output (e.g. based on significant correlation). Other methods consider combinations of variables in a heuristic manner, for example, forward, backward, and mixed stepwise selections. In forward selection, input variables are added one-at-a-time to a model containing no input variables. The variable that improves model performance the most is added at each step, until a predetermined performance threshold is reached (e.g. AIC of x is "good enough"). In essence, this allows choosing the smallest model with a predetermined acceptable model performance threshold. Backward stepwise selection follows similar steps, except the initial model is one containing all candidate input variables, and the least useful input variable is removed sequentially until a performance threshold is reached. Mixed stepwise selection combines forward and backward selection.

Conversely, **dimension reduction** (or dimensionality reduction) *transforms* potential input variables into a set of fewer surrogate variables (lower dimensions). For example, dimension reduction may narrow the aforementioned list of candidate input variables to three variables (var_1, var_2, var_3). These reduced dimensions may be interpretable, e.g. var_1 may still represent age, var_2 may be derived from a combination of (*co-morbidity A, co_morbidity B*) and var_3 from (*disease A, disease B*). However, generally, the features derived through dimensionality reduction are not necessarily interpretable and may represent rather complex concepts.

While feature selection considers the outcome (i.e. supervised), dimension reduction generally does not (i.e. unsupervised).

12.2.7 Performance Metrics

We have alluded to model performance in the preceding sections: what is an optimal algorithm? How can we assess whether the algorithm is performing well? There are several ways to assess model performance. We will discuss the most common metrics.

For **classification**, most are familiar with the 2 × 2 table of predicted vs. actual results (true positive/negative, false positive/negative) which derive sensitivity, specificity, positive predictive value, and negative predictive value. In machine learning terminology, this 2 × 2 table is called the *confusion matrix.*

There are several synonyms to be familiar with. "**Precision**" is a synonym for positive predictive value (PPV), while "**recall**" is a synonym for sensitivity. Both are commonly reported performance metrics for algorithms. A model with high precision is favorable when the cost of false positives is high (e.g. if a positive result would lead to an invasive intervention). A model with high recall (or positive predictive value) is favorable when the cost of false negative is high (e.g. septic shock prediction). Precision (or PPV) can be defined in two variants. In its first common variant, precision is the ratio of true positives over the number of predicted positives. The second variant is applied in case–control studies where prevalence in the overall population is taken into account. For example, an algorithm with 99% sensitivity and 99% specificity to detect SMA syndrome will have low PPV if the prevalence of SMA syndrome in the overall population is low. "F1 **score**," the harmonic mean of precision and recall

$$F1 = \frac{(2 \times \text{precision} \times \text{recall})}{(\text{precision} + \text{recall})}$$

is another commonly reported model metric.

Accuracy is also derived from the confusion matrix and reflects the total proportion of correctly classified subjects (true positives and true negatives). Accuracy may not be an informative metric when the dataset has heavy class imbalance (e.g. many negatives and few positives). For example, consider an algorithm that aims to classify patients with and without ischemic bowel. If only ten subjects among 1000 have ischemic bowel, yet the algorithm always predicts that a patient does not have ischemic bowel, this algorithm would have 99% accuracy despite incorrectly classifying all patients who do have ischemic bowel.

Area under the receiver-operator curve (**AUROC**) is another commonly reported metric. AUROC ranges from 0 to 1 and reflects a model's discrimination capacity. Understanding AUROC requires thorough understanding of several concepts. First, classification algorithms can return predictions on a continuous scale (often interpreted but not always equivalent to class probabilities). And, discrimination ability of that continuous output is reflected by how well these values can distinguish different classes (for example, binary or categorical outcome labels). Since the output of the model is continuous, thresholds have to be chosen for making a final decision about the predicted class. Second, AUROC reflects the trade-off between true positive rate (sensitivity) and false-positive rate (1 − specificity) across all possible thresholds. The receiver-operator curve (the ROC in AUROC) is represented on a graph where the y-axis reflects true positive rates, and the x-axis reflects false-positive rates as the classification threshold is varied. Thus, different points on the curve reflect different thresholds for separating two classes (e.g. diseased vs. non-diseased). As the threshold to belong to the "diseased" class decreases, the sensitivity increases, while the specificity decreases (if an algorithm classifies all subjects as positive [low threshold], the sensitivity would be 100%). The ROC curve can be thought of as a series of points that reflects varying model sensitivity and specificity with threshold changes (near the origin reflects the highest threshold, near the top-right corner reflects the lowest threshold). The AUROC is a singular value summarizing sensitivities–specificities across different model thresholds and can be interpreted as the probability that if a positive and negative sample were chosen at random, the positive sample would be correctly ranked as more likely to be positive than the negative sample. For example, AUROC of 1 would mean all patients with a disease were ranked as having higher probability of being in the "diseased" class than patients without the disease. Of note, AUROC values sensitivity and specificity equally, which may be inappropriate for many clinical applications.

Area under the precision recall curve (**AUPRC**) is similar to AUROC, but may be a more informative performance metric when accurately identifying positives is important or when the dataset is heavily imbalanced. The AUPRC has the same conceptual idea as AUROC, except that the x-axis reflects recall (positive predictive value) rather than 1 − sensitivity (true negative rate). While the AUROC of a random classifier (e.g. coin flip) is 0.5, the AUPRC of a random classifier is the proportion of positives in the population. The AUPRC ranges from 0 to 1. If a model achieves perfect AUPRC (1), this would mean all positives were classified as positives without accidentally labeling negatives as positive.

For **regression**, the most common performance metric is the mean squared error (**MSE**). The MSE quantifies how close the predicted value for a particular observation is to the true value of that observation by averaging the sum of squared differences between the predicted and observed outcome values. The root mean squared error (**RMSE**) is an extension of the MSE, found by taking the square root of the MSE (not the average of sum of root mean squared errors). An advantage of RMSE over MSE is that the units equal those of the outcome. Mean absolute error (MAE) is a similar metric to quantify how closely predicted outcomes match observed outcomes, by averaging the sum of absolute differences between predicted and observed outcome values. The residual standard error (**RSE**) and the R^2 are two other common metrics to evaluate accuracy of linear regression models. RSE is positively correlated with the residual sum of squares (**RSS**); small RSE suggests the algorithm fits the data well. The R^2, ranging from 0 to 1, quantifies the proportion of outcome variability that can be explained by model inputs. For example, R^2 value of 1 would indicate that all changes in the outcome can be fully explained by changes in the algorithm's input variable values. A higher R^2 is more favorable.

12.2.8 Training, Validation, and Test Sets

Algorithms will perform best on samples they have already seen, i.e. on the dataset they were built and trained on. But the crucible of an algorithm's clinical utility is its performance "in the real world," i.e. its *generalizability*. Without performing expensive multi-center studies, how can we assess how an algorithm may perform "in the real world"?

For this, we can evaluate algorithm performance on a dataset distinct from the one it was built on. Before building an algorithm, the available data can be divided into training and test sets. The training set, sometimes called the "development set," is used to build and optimize the algorithm. This includes, for example, selecting the right algorithm and tuning hyperparameters. After the development phase, the constructed algorithm is applied to a test set that was kept separately (no test set subject should inform algorithm development). The model performance on this test set then may suggest possible performance in clinical scenarios. This approach is called the ***holdout method***.

In almost all cases, test set performance will be worse than training set performance; this is expected, because by definition, machine learning algorithms are *trained* using the training set, i.e. during the training phase the algorithm has seen the corresponding samples. In contrast the samples in the test are novel to the algorithm. If there is a considerable gap between training and test set performance, this may indicate model overfitting. If there is little gap between training and test set performance, and the performance in both sets is poor, this may indicate model underfitting (the model did not "learn" well).

To ensure applicability to real-world scenarios, it is important to appropriately choose the training and test set. In particular, it should avoid a so-called **selection bias** (of particular individuals or groups) by reflecting the characteristics of the population the algorithm is applied to in practice. For example, both training and test sets should contain an appropriate proportion of positive and negative samples, have patients with similar overall distribution of input variable values, account for possible demographic biases and temporal shifts, etc. Traditionally, the training set comprises a higher proportion of the data than the test set (e.g. 80:20 split, 70:30 split). However, some in the machine learning community would argue that the test set should be larger, as larger test sets more accurately reflect expected model performance in real-world scenarios. Conversely, increasing the test set size reduces the number of samples in the training set and as such the number of samples the algorithm can train on which may result in models with lower predictive power. Thus, there is no golden rule for a ratio that should determine training and test set splits. When the train-test ratio is set, in practice, data is often split randomly which is appropriate for large datasets where we assume that the characteristics of the target population are well represented. If datasets are smaller, stratified sampling strategies are employed that explicitly balance target variables, and in some cases also various other population characteristics. Of note, "randomness" in most statistical software is not truly random, but follows patterns determined by preset "seeds". Thus, to ensure replicability during model development, the random seed number can be encoded (e.g. seed "15") before performing train-test splits.

During development it can be useful to estimate the performance of an algorithm on unseen data, in order to estimate and optimize generalizability. For this, since it is important to not use metrics and statistics on the test set to develop and tune algorithms, a proportion of the training set is often used as a separate *validation dataset,* resulting in a three-way spit of the data: a **training dataset** (excluding the validation dataset), the **validation dataset** (split from the training set), and the **test dataset**. During development, the validation dataset is not used for training the algorithm, and, thus, evaluating the resulting model on the validation dataset gives an estimate of how the algorithm will perform on unseen samples. This enables better refinement of the algorithm by preventing overfitting and optimizing generalizability, without employing the test set. Note that in machine learning research, the test set is sometimes called a "validation set," particularly if the data is only split into two subsets, i.e. a training and a test/validation dataset. The three-way split is most often seen in the deep learning context (see Sect. 12.3.4) where large datasets are most prevalent.

12.2.8.1 Cross-Validation

The previous section considers a single split into training (validation) and test set in order to estimate the performance of the trained algorithm in real-world applications, i.e. its generalizability on unseen data. As only a single split is evaluated, the estimated performance may be dependent on the particular split that has been chosen and thus may not accurately reflect the actual performance. To prevent this, the general notion of **cross-validation** [1] consists of repeatedly splitting the data into train and test splits and calculating an aggregate performance metric across these splits. For this, cross-validation comprises several techniques to split the dataset into training and test sets (e.g. leave-one-out cross-validation, k-fold cross-validation). A common variant is *k-fold cross-validation*. For example, for tenfold cross-validation, the dataset is split into ten "folds." This results in ten steps, one for each of the ten folds. In each step, the corresponding fold is used as a test set and the nine remaining folds are used as the training set. The model is then trained on this training set and the performance metric is evaluated on the corresponding test set (similar to the previously introduced holdout method). This is repeated for each fold and an average of the performance metric over all folds is reported. As the final performance metric is an average over multiple data splits with different training and test sets, cross-validation is expected to give a better estimate of the generalization capabilities of the algorithm. Commonly, the mean and standard deviation of the performance metric across folds are reported.

Variants There are multiple variants of cross-validation. For example, in ***leave-one-out cross-validation***, the dataset is split by sample. That is, one sample is left out and the model is trained on all the remaining samples. Consequently, there are as many folds as there are samples. As such, leave-one-out cross-validation is an *exhaustive* cross-validation scheme, as all possible testing sets with a single sample contribute to the final performance metric. In contrast, k-fold cross-validation is *non-exhaustive* as the k folds can be arbitrarily chosen. To make sure that a particular split into folds does not randomly return a particular good or bad performance, it is also common to employ *repeated k-fold cross-validation* which refers to repeating k-fold cross-validation with different splits in order to get a better estimate of the performance metric across these splits. Finally, ***nested cross-validation*** refers to first splitting the data into multiple training and test splits as for the previous cases. This first step is referred to as the outer *cross-validation layer*. Then for each split, another layer of cross-validation is used during training, referred to as the *inner layer.* This inner layer is used to optimize the corresponding model, e.g. using hyperparameter tuning or variable selection. This can make the trained models more generalizable with regard to the performance in the outer layer.

Practical Considerations While cross-validation can yield more robust performance estimates than the holdout method, it is not always straightforward or appropriate to apply. For example, in cases where the data may contain duplicates or very similar samples, cross-validation may return too optimistic performance estimates. Also, in cases with large discrepancies in the number of cases and controls, stratified cross-validation has to be employed to keep the case/control ratio consistent between training and test sets. Similarly, it may be necessary to ensure that particular groups of samples, e.g. with regard to demographics or sites, are equally distributed between training and test splits to avoid bias. Additionally, in cases where the data changes over time, it may make more sense to employ a holdout approach, where we split the data into older data points for training and newer data points for testing in order to measure the generalizability of the model across time. A similar scenario may be applicable for a study spanning multiple study sites. Thus, it is important to keep in mind which aspect of a model we want to test and whether cross-validation measures this aspect appropriately.

Finally, it is important to note that models must not be iteratively optimized based on cross-validation scores, particularly if that score is the only reported performance metric. That is, while the likelihood of overfitting is decreased, by iteratively adjusting models based on a cross-validation score the model is still likely to be overfitted on that data. This likely causes too optimistic performance estimates as well as a poor performance on an unseen test dataset. To cope with this, either the models and their parameters have to be chosen beforehand without involving the data and only then be evaluated via cross-validation. Or the performance on a completely separate test set (often referred to as validation set in this context) should be reported. Optimally, if comparability permits, such a separate test set is obtained from a different source than the previous dataset used for cross-validation. Note that cross-validation does not yield a single best model, but trains a different model for each fold (e.g. with different feature importances). As such, to apply the model to the separate test set, the model is usually trained again on the complete dataset previously used for cross-validation.

12.3 Evolution of a Family of Machine Learning Algorithms: From Linear Models to Deep Learning

We have discussed several fundamental concepts applicable to many machine learning algorithms. This section will provide a practical introduction to common machine learning algorithms following the natural progression from logistic and linear regression to deep learning models. We skip algorithms like support vector machines, decision trees, as well as meta learners like ensemble or boosting methods and point the reader to appropriate literature [2].

12.3.1 Supervised Learning

This chapter will discuss supervised machine learning algorithms. In supervised learning, the outcome variable is *predefined* by the researcher, and the algorithm aims to map input variables to the outcome variable. Conversely, in unsupervised learning, there is no predefined outcome variable. Unsupervised learning algorithms aim to explore relationships between individual variables or subjects, rather than mapping how to get from input variables to a predefined output variable. Semi-supervised learning refers to cases where output variables are only available for a subset of the training data.

12.3.2 Logistic and Linear Regression

Logistic regression is a supervised machine learning algorithm for classification problems. Classification problems address how inputs can be mapped to categorical outputs (classes). For example, the research question, "is there an association between acute cholecystitis Tokyo grade and 30-day mortality," has a binary output (30-day mortality: yes or no). Logistic regression is one of the most commonly used methods in surgical health services research. Many surgeons are likely familiar with the concept of odds ratios and 95% confidence intervals. But what exactly is the logistic regression algorithm doing?

Logistic regression algorithms model the probability the outcome belongs in a particular class (e.g. "diseased" class). This probability can be converted to odds by the formula,

$$\mathbf{odds} = \frac{\text{probability}}{1 - \text{probability:}}$$

odds thus range from 0 to infinity.

When a logistic regression is built using a statistical program, the researcher will write code such as (outcome ~ input_variable$_1$ + input_variable$_2$ + …input_variable$_n$). The program will usually output β coefficients for the intercept and each input variable, such as $\beta_{\text{intercept}}$, β_1, β_2, ... β_n. Specifically, logistic regression with more than one input variable (here n variables) is called multiple or multivariable logistic regression. Of note, this is different from multivariate logistic regression, which refers to regression models with more than one output variable. The β coefficients can be transformed into odds ratios by exponentiation (e.g. e^{β}). A negative β coefficient will translate to odds ratios <1, while a positive β coefficient will translate to odds ratios >1. The "O" odds ratio for a specific input variable, e.g. input_variable_*i*, in a multivariable logistic regression model can be interpreted as, "holding all other input variables constant, a 1-unit increase in input_variable_1 will translate to O change in odds of the outcome." Of note, the "unit" refers to the scale under which input variable data entered the model; if "weight" was entered in kg, the unit would be kg, and if weight was entered as g, the unit would be g.

Linear regression is a supervised machine learning algorithm for quantitative prediction problems (i.e. continuous outcome variable). Similar to logistic regression, linear regression entails the equation, outcome $y = \beta\_\text{intercept} + \beta_1 \times \text{input\_variable}_1 + \ldots\beta_n \times \text{input\_variable}_n$. Linear regression models most commonly choose β coefficients that minimize the *residual sum of squares (**RSS**)*, which is the sum of squares of errors between the predicted and the actual outcomes at every given input-output pair. As with any machine learning algorithm, the linear relationship between the inputs and the output is derived from incomplete data, yet seeks to model the relationship in the real world. The "**standard error**" (square root of the sample mean's variance) estimates the average amount the estimated output from incomplete data differs from the population output and is inversely proportional with sample size. The standard error is used to calculate 95% confidence intervals for β coefficients and for hypothesis testing. If an estimated β coefficient is far enough from zero (distance as determined by standard error of the β coefficient), the associated p value would be small and suggest our data is incompatible with the null hypothesis (there is no significant difference between specified populations).

Significance of regression coefficients: Many researchers building multiple regression may be tempted to look at p values associated with each β coefficient and conclude that those with p values <0.05 are "significant predictors of the outcome." This is a common fallacy. Numerous misinterpretations of p values have resulted in improper inferences being drawn from logistic regression and other models. A p value is *not* the probability that the study hypothesis is true (e.g. "a difference exists between group A and B"), nor is it the probability that the results were produced by random chance alone. In hypothesis testing, the p value can be thought of as the probability of achieving a more extreme value than the one from the model. In other words, rather than a statement about the hypothesis, the p value is a statement about the data in relation to a hypothesis: the smaller the p value, the more incompatible the data is with the null hypothesis. The 0.05 threshold is a relatively arbitrary threshold commonly used in surgical literature; some epidemiologists argue for lowering the threshold of significance to 0.005! It is important to note that p values depend on three factors: the effect size, sample size, and measurement precision. If the population size is large enough, despite little difference in effect size (e.g. evaluating the effect of injury severity score on mortality, group A had ISS of 14 vs. group B had ISS of 13, p value was 0.03), the p value may be small. Thus, statistical significance does not equal clinical significance. Moreover, if enough input variables are included within a model, some input variables' p values will be <0.05 by chance. For example, if 100 variables that have absolutely no association with an outcome are included in a model predicting an outcome, the p values for approximately 5 of those variables would be <0.05 by chance alone. In summary, no scientific or clinical decisions should be made solely on the basis of a p value threshold.

Feature interaction and selection for regression models: A research hypothesis usually assumes that an input variable x is associated with output y, yet several other covariates are included in the multiple regression model. If p values alone should not inform variable selection for model inference, how should we choose which variables to include in the multiple logistic regression model? Before considering available options, we note that different disciplines refer to these non-primary input variables as covariates or confounders. Some disciplines distinguish these two terms, but in practice, **covariates** and **confounders** are interchangeable terms when used as input variables. Confounders are associated with both the main predictor and the outcome (but not in the causal pathway). Some non-primary variables may be "**moderators**," which change the magnitude of the relationship between the predictor and the outcome. Moderators are coded in most statistical programs in the format, outcome ~ predictor × moderator. "**Effect modifiers**" and "**interaction terms**" are synonyms for moderators.

Criteria for selecting variables to use in a multiple logistic regression model should be determined a priori before conducting analysis. Two general criteria for selecting variables are clinical and statistical. Clinical criteria, or the "sanity check," entails selecting covariates that reasonably confound or moderate the association between the predictor and outcome, e.g. based on domain knowledge. A common statistical criteria may include decision based on how many data points have valid values as large amounts of missing data make predictions challenging. Evaluating different combinations of input variables that result in the most "significant" outcome (e.g. highest odds ratio, lowest p value ["p-hacking"]) is scientifically invalid and may only be applied on data that is not used in the final study. In addition to these criteria, it is possible to integrate variable selection into the training process strictly excluding any samples from the data that is used to derive the model performance from. Several variable selection and dimensionality reduction techniques are discussed in Sect. 12.2.6. Furthermore, a regression specific method is to base variable selection (within the training step) on including covariates that change the β coefficient of the main predictor in univariate analysis by a predetermined threshold (e.g. 20%). For example, if the β coefficient of the main predictor in the univariate regression, outcome ~ predictor is 0.3, but this β coefficient increases to 0.4 (33% change) in the regression, outcome ~ predictor + covariate, this covariate would be included in the final algorithm. Other considerations and strategies for variable selection (must be performed during training), such as multicollinearity and regularization, will be discussed in the next section.

Regularization: Regularization techniques can be applied to both logistic and linear regression to mitigate overfitting or address multicollinearity. *Lasso* (L1) regularization is in essence a variable selection technique developed for logistic and linear regression which is integrated into the training process. Conceptually, regularization adds a penalty term to decrease the value of β coefficients in regression models towards (**Ridge**, or L2 regularization) or to (**Lasso**, or L1 regularization) zero. Decreasing a β coefficient value reduces the impact the associated input variable has in determining the outcome. Unlike Ridge regularization, Lasso regularization can reduce some β coefficients to zero; this removes certain input variables from the algorithm (multiplying by a zero coefficient cancels out the input variable value). In essence, L1 regularization helps identify the most important input variables that are associated with the output variable.

Ridge (L2) regularization is not a variable selection technique (does not reduce the number of input variables), but is helpful for addressing **multicollinearity**, another important concept to consider for multiple regression models. Multicollinearity occurs when input variables are correlated with each other. For example, a model containing both weight and body mass index will have multicollinearity. Multicollinearity introduces multiple problems for regression models. In brief, multicollinearity makes model coefficients unstable (coefficients can vary widely and even change signs depending on which other input variables are included) and inflates standard errors of coefficients, which subsequently weakens statistical power of the algorithm (ability to detect a difference when a true difference exists). The most common way to detect multicollinearity in a model is by calculating the variance inflation factor (**VIF**) for each input variable in the model. Higher VIF (common thresholds include 5 or 10) suggests greater concern for multicollinearity with other input variables in the model. Variable selection is one way to address multicollinearity. Without delving into mathematical details, ridge regularization helps address multicollinearity by estimating more precise β coefficients.

For both Lasso and Ridge regularization, how much β coefficient values are reduced is determined by **λ** (***lambda***), a hyperparameter (see previous introduction of models, Sect. 12.2.1). For example, higher lambda values will reduce β coefficients of regression models further and lead to less flexible models (lower variance, higher bias). Like any hyperparameter, lambda values can be tuned, in order to find the model with the best combinations of coefficients resulting in the highest model performance (best bias-variance tradeoff). Note that this optimization has to occur on the training data only, without considering the performance on the test data.

12.3.3 Generalized Additive Models

Generalized additive models (**GAM**) are supervised machine learning algorithms that can be used for both categorical and continuous outcomes. The previous section detailed several strategies to fine-tune linear regression algorithms. Despite using regularization or other techniques, linear regression algorithms are limited by the linearity assumption. For some research questions, it may not be impossible to map any combination of inputs linearly to an output. Conceptually, GAM replace each multiplication with a β coefficient in a linear model with a unique non-linear function f [outcome ~ f_1(input_variable$_1$) + f_2(input_variable$_2$)… + f_n(input_variable$_n$)]. GAM allow more complex relationships between input variables and output to be mapped more accurately while maintaining model interpretability (the effect of each input variable on the outcome is defined by its responsible function). Including non-linear functions yields more complex algorithms that decrease variance while increasing bias.

There are several strategies to build non-linear functions. A simple strategy is to include polynomial input variables (e.g. x^n, where $n > 1$) within the function (*polynomial function*). Beyond polynomial functions, other non-linear functions include step functions and splines. **Step functions** entail converting a continuous input variable into categories and applying different functions to different category values. For example, if age is the input variable of interest, a step function may comprise one function to compute an outcome from ages <18 years (e.g. outcome = age × 2) and another function to compute the same outcome from ages >18 years (e.g. outcome = age × 3 + 5). **Splines** combine polynomial and step functions. Spline functions apply different polynomial functions to different ranges of continuous input values. **Splines** "smooth out" the curves built by different functions, allowing a continuous, non-linear curve to define the association between an input variable and the outcome at all ranges of input variable values. "**Knots**" indicate threshold input variable values where polynomial functions change; statistical programs can automate select the optimal location and number of knots to derive the most optimal splines.

12.3.4 Deep Learning

Deep learning models extend the capabilities of the previously mentioned models by allowing to fit more complex (theoretically arbitrary), non-linear relationships between input variables and the output of interest. In theory this can produce more powerful models and allows to incorporate data beyond the previously discussed tabular format. More complex data formats include, for example, images, text, or time series and even arbitrary combinations. However, while it has been shown that deep learning models can yield powerful models that may achieve superhuman performance, for example, in the context of image recognition, [3] deep learning models often require large amounts of training data and careful engineering to perform well, and the resulting predictions are often hard to interpret. In the following, we give a brief overview of the terminology and anatomy of deep learning models, highlight their flexibility, and discuss the considerations that are important for their application in practice. Note that we concentrate on supervised learning and predictive models rather than giving an exhaustive overview of all deep learning architectures and variants [4, 5].

Basic terminology: The term "deep learning" summarizes models that are based on simplistic computational approximations of neural networks, also called *artificial neural networks (ANN)*. The term "deep learning model" and "(artificial) neural network" are often used interchangeably. In their most simple form (called *multi-layer perceptrons* or *MLPs*), these neural networks are made up of a sequence of connected layers which in turn consist of a set of individual neurons. The first layer is called the *input layer*, the last layer is called the *output layer*. Input variables are mapped to neurons in the input layer, then information sequentially passes from the input layer through all layers, until the neurons in the output layer represent the output or prediction of the neural network. Historically, a neural network is called a "deep" neural network if the number of layers is sufficiently large. However, in practice, often any neural network architecture is referred to as a deep learning model regardless of its complexity.

Anatomy: On a more detailed level, each layer of a neural network contains a set of neurons. In a standard multi-layer perceptron (MLP), all neurons of two subsequent layers are connected to each other, while neurons within a layer are not connected. Through these connections, neurons in each predecessor layer can "activate" neurons in their subsequent layer. This sequentially propagates the signals provided by the input variables from the input layer to the output layer which then represents the predictions of the network. The activation of a single neuron is calculated through **activation functions** (commonly non-linear) that map a set of input signals of neurons from the preceding layer to an output signal for that neuron. The input signals of a neuron are weighted. These ***weights*** represent the ***model*** parameters of the neural network and allow it to learn the relationship between input variables and the desired output. The power of neural networks lies in their flexibility of how layers are designed, and how the previously described propagation of signals activates neurons from layer to layer.

Examples: In their simplest form, neural networks map the input layer with n input variables directly to an output layer with only a single output neuron using a linear activation function. Mathematically, this can be represented as $y = \beta_0 + \beta_1 \times x_1 + \ldots \beta_n \times x_n$, where β_0 is a learnable intercept weight, β_i are weights for each input neuron, and x_i are the values of the input variables. Notably, this simple neural network is equivalent to linear regression discussed above. More advanced instances introduce additional layers, non-linear activation functions, more complex connectivity profiles, and more. Concrete examples are, convolution neural networks, [6] used for visual tasks like image annotation or video analysis, which mimic the biological design of the visual system, and reuse particular layers across the neural network and the visual input. Another extension are recurrent neural networks, which allow layers to propagate their signal back to preceding layers which enables the processing of sequences like text or continuously measured biological signals. These are just two relatively simple examples of deep learning models, and current deep learning research aims at finding the right architectures based on different tasks and the available data. Note that for some applications, recent deep learning models consist of billions of neurons and take months and millions of dollars to train [7].

Training: Generally, neural networks are trained in an iterative manner. Each step is called an ***epoch***. In each epoch the training data is split into ***batches***. For each batch, the neural network is then applied to the corresponding subset of training data in what is called a *forward pass*. Then a ***loss function*** is applied to calculate a *loss* which specifies how well the neural network performs on that batch (for example, the mean squared error to the desired outcome). This loss is then used to update the weights of the neural network in a so-called *backward pass*. The process by which this is achieved is called ***back-propagation***, as the loss flows backward from the model output to the input. The degree of change throughout the network based on this loss is regulated by an ***optimizer*** and often a corresponding *learning rate*. This is done for each batch in an epoch and then repeated for several epochs. The optimizer, learning rate, the number of batches and epochs, and generally the learning process can be intricate to tune and have a large influence on the performance of the model. In particular, overfitting and underfitting are a more prevalent issue than for other approaches. For this reason, in most cases, training deep learning models is done using a training, validation, test split (see Sect. 12.2.8 on Training and Validation), where the training set is used for training the current configuration, and the performance of the model is carefully monitored on the validation set to optimize the model and training procedure. Only after this is done, the test set is used to evaluate the final performance of the model. Using this three-way split ensures a stable training procedure and prevents overfitting on the test data but required relatively large datasets.

Considerations for the application of deep learning: While deep learning has the potential to outperform simpler approaches, designing and training deep learning models can be challenging. First, due to their inherent flexibility and the ensuing plethora of model variants, the number of hyperparameters to tune in order for deep learning models to perform well is extraordinarily large. Similarly, the training process described previously can be challenging to tune. Thus, often, in-depth knowledge on the behavior of different aspects of neural networks is necessary to train well-performing models. Furthermore, due to the flexibility of neural networks and their capabilities to learn complex relationships, they need more data to train than simpler models like linear regression depending on the application and complexity of the model. Current state-of-the-art models train on millions of training samples [8]. Nevertheless, while deep learning models only recently can compete with more common machine learning models on tabular data [9], the particular strength of deep learning lies in directly working on complex data without the need of laborious preprocessing. This also enables deep learning models to discover unknown features of the data that may be informative for a given task and have previously not been discovered. However, this process may also lead deep learning models to find "spurious shortcuts" rather than actual signals in the data [10]. Furthermore, in the context of multi-modal learning [11], deep learning models can directly train on a combination of input modalities simultaneously, e.g. image data, videos or audio, allowing them to integrate information that was previously hard to combine. For example, medical imaging pixel-based models may integrate contextual data from electronic health records [12]. Furthermore, in the context of multi-task learning [13], deep learning models are able to improve their performance by predicting several outcomes at the same time inherently exploiting the underlying relation of the corresponding tasks. Finally, while deep learning approaches can yield powerful models, an important consideration for applying neural networks is their inherent lack of interpretability. While current research aims at alleviating this issue [14], generally, deep learning models learn complex relationships and thus their predictions are often hard to explain.

Overall, deep learning models are a powerful tool to train models that can achieve superhuman performance particularly as advancement in technology and monitoring systems allows for large amounts of data to be collected and stored. However their design, training, and interpretation is a challenging and potentially time consuming process that has to be taken into account when applying deep learning in practice.

Acknowledgements This work was supported by the American Heart Association (19PABHI34580007), Burroughs Wellcome Fund (1019816), NIH (1R61NS114926), and NIH (R35GM138353).

References

1. King RD, Orhobor OI, Taylor CC. Cross-validation is safe to use. Nat Mach Intell. 2021;3(4):276. https://doi.org/10.1038/s42256-021-00332-z.
2. Alpaydin E. Introduction to machine learning. 4th ed. Cambridge, MA: MIT Press; 2020.
3. Cireşan D, Meier U, Masci J, Schmidhuber J. Multi-column deep neural network for traffic sign classification. Neural Netw. 2012;32:333–8. https://doi.org/10.1016/j.neunet.2012.02.023.
4. Alzubaidi L, Zhang J, Humaidi AJ, Al-Dujaili A, Duan Y, Al-Shamma O, Santamaría J, Fadhel MA, Al-Amidie M, Farhan L. Review of deep learning: concepts, CNN architectures, challenges, applications, future directions. J Big Data. 2021;8(1):53. https://doi.org/10.1186/s40537-021-00444-8.
5. Liu W, Wang Z, Liu X, Zeng N, Liu Y, Alsaadi FE. A survey of deep neural network architectures and their applications. Neurocomputing. 2017;234:11–26. https://doi.org/10.1016/j.neucom.2016.12.038.
6. Yamashita R, Nishio M, Do RKG, Togashi K. Convolutional neural networks: an overview and application in radiology. Insights Imaging. 2018;9(4):611–29. https://doi.org/10.1007/s13244-018-0639-9.
7. Brown TB, Mann B, Ryder N, Subbiah M, Kaplan J, Dhariwal P, Neelakantan A, Shyam P, Sastry G, Askell A, et al. Language models are few-shot learners. ArXiv200514165 Cs. 2020. http://arxiv.org/abs/2005.14165. Accessed 3 Dec 2021.
8. Gorban AN, Makarov VA, Tyukin IY. The unreasonable effectiveness of small neural ensembles in high-dimensional brain. Phys Life Rev. 2019;29:55–88. https://doi.org/10.1016/j.plrev.2018.09.005.
9. Arik SÖ, Pfister T. TabNet: attentive interpretable tabular learning. Proc AAAI Conf Artif Intell. 2021;35(8):6679–87.
10. DeGrave AJ, Janizek JD, Lee S-I. AI for radiographic COVID-19 detection selects shortcuts over signal. Nat Mach Intell. 2021;3(7):610–9. https://doi.org/10.1038/s42256-021-00338-7.
11. Ngiam J, Khosla A, Kim M, Nam J, Lee H, Ng AY. Multimodal deep learning. In: Proceedings of the 28th International Conference on International Conference on Machine Learning. ICML'11. Madison, WI: Omnipress; 2011.
12. Huang S-C, Pareek A, Seyyedi S, Banerjee I, Lungren MP. Fusion of medical imaging and electronic health records using deep learning: a systematic review and implementation guidelines. NPJ Digit Med. 2020;3(1):1–9. https://doi.org/10.1038/s41746-020-00341-z.
13. Ruder S. An overview of multi-task learning in deep neural networks. ArXiv170605098 Cs Stat. 2017. http://arxiv.org/abs/1706.05098. Accessed 3 Dec 2021.
14. Barredo Arrieta A, Díaz-Rodríguez N, Del Ser J, Bennetot A, Tabik S, Barbado A, Garcia S, Gil-Lopez S, Molina D, Benjamins R, et al. Explainable Artificial Intelligence (XAI): concepts, taxonomies, opportunities and challenges toward responsible AI. Inf Fusion. 2020;58:82–115. https://doi.org/10.1016/j.inffus.2019.12.012.

Statistical Editor's Practical Advice for Data Analysis

13

Fikri M. Abu-Zidan

13.1 Introduction

Working as a Statistical Editor for international refereed journals for the last 20 years, I find that the majority of serious statistical errors are easy to avoid if the authors take care to follow very basic principles. I hope that this can be achieved if attention is taken when reading this short chapter. I will mainly address the basic statistical analysis when performed by young researchers. I advise readers who are not experts in statistics and want to perform advanced statistical methods like logistic regression, mixed linear models, or general linear models to consult and follow the advice of an experienced statistician. These models require specific assumptions that have to be fulfilled to be reliable [1]. Nevertheless, the majority of basic univariate analysis can be performed with confidence following the recommendations given in this chapter.

Learning Objectives

- Understand the importance of building the analysis based on the research question.
- Simplify the theoretical background to justify the selection of the analysis.
- Enable the reader to define the rules in which he/she can select the proper statistical method.
- Have a practical map that can direct the analysis process.
- Enforce the learning process through practical applications.

F. M. Abu-Zidan (✉)
The Research Office, College of Medicine and Health, Sciences, United Arab Emirates University, Al-Ain, United Arab Emirates

M. Ceresoli et al. (eds.), *Statistics and Research Methods for Acute Care and General Surgeons*, Hot Topics in Acute Care Surgery and Trauma,
https://doi.org/10.1007/978-3-031-13818-8_13

Table 13.1 Basic questions to be answered before starting the analysis

Sequence	Question
Question 1	What is the objective of the analysis?
Question 2	What is the type of data?
Question 3	Are the data normally distributed?
Question 4	How many groups are compared? (two or more than two)
Question 5	What is the number of subjects in each group?
Question 6	Are the compared data related or unrelated?

There are six questions that have to be answered in sequence before starting the analysis. These are shown in Table 13.1. If answered properly, I hope that the correct statistical methods will be selected. We will go through these questions in sequence.

13.2 What Is the Objective of the Analysis?

Statistics is only a tool to summarize and compare data in an informative way. It is essential to define the research question and the objectives of the analysis before even starting it. This is more important when analyzing data retrieved from retrospective studies or large clinical registries. Statistics cannot salvage an inadequate research question or poorly designed study.

Simple descriptive statistics can sometimes be sufficient in high-quality research projects. Collaborators who approach me to perform an advanced statistical analysis get occasionally surprised to see that I used simple descriptive statistics instead of comparative statistical methods because that could address the aim of the study [2]. Statistics is simply a tool to answer the research question, not an aim by itself. Furthermore, the quality of the analysis will depend on the quality of the data. Never start any statistical analysis before getting assured that the data is of good quality and properly coded. If the objective is well defined, the data is accurate, well-understood, and properly coded, you will be surprised to see how the statistical analysis is easy, smooth, and straightforward. The results should then be accepted regardless of the outcome. I personally aim to perform the statistical analysis only once and accept its results even if they were negative.

Unfortunately, it is a common practice that some researchers perform repeated subgroup analysis, fishing for a significant *p* value and then retrospectively define the research question to fit the data after the analysis. This is usually difficult to detect. It is erroneous, non-professional, and may even be a research misconduct if not explicitly mentioned in the methods. A clear example for that is the interim analysis of randomized controlled trials, if not declared, which should be transparent as part of the research protocol. It is more difficult in retrospective studies to know whether the results were hypothesis-driven with

Table 13.2 Mechanism of injury of hospitalized patients involved with road traffic collisions during the pre-COVID-19 and COVID-19 periods, Al-Ain City, United Arab Emirates

Variable	Pre-COVID period $n = 750$	COVID period $n = 499$	*P* value
Mechanism of injury			<0.0001
Motor vehicle collision	540 (72)	302 (60.5)	
Motorcycle	84 (11.2)	116 (23.3)	
Bicycle	42 (5.6)	35 (7)	
Pedestrian	84 (11.2)	46 (9.2)	

a clear research question to be answered or whether they stemmed from fishing for a *p* value [3]. This will depend on the conscious and integrity of the researcher.

Table 13.2 gives an example of how defining the research question clearly makes the statistical analysis focused. It shows the mechanism of road traffic collisions in Al-Ain City, United Arab Emirates, before and after the COVID-19 pandemic in one of our recently published papers [4]. The analysis in this scenario will depend on the research question. If the question is: "Is there difference in the mechanism of injury of road traffic collisions before and during the COVID-19 Pandemic?" then Pearson's Chi-Square test using a 4×2 table should be used. This will produce only a single *p* value. The subgroup analysis comparing each mechanism alone between the two groups will increase the chance of getting significance by multiple testing. This will include four comparisons, each with a type I error of 5% of finding statistical significance by chance. Multiple testing can be done as post hoc analysis to explain the significance but not to prove it. If the overall analysis was not significant, then the post hoc analysis should not be performed.

Understandably, the probability of finding statistical significance by chance increases with each additional subgroup analysis [3]. Bonferroni correction can be used to protect against this error by defining the proper *p* value to be 0.05 divided by the number of subgroup pair comparisons [5].

13.3 What Is the Type of Data?

The second step is to thoroughly understand the nature and type of the studied variables (Table 13.3). *Categorical (nominal) data* (like eye color or race) do not have an ordered nature nor a measurement of distance between different categories. Even if categorical data are numbered during statistical analysis, these numbers are artificial and just represent the category [6]. *Binary data* is a special type of categorical data that has only two possible options. These are mutually exclusive where one option implies the negation of the other (like dead and alive). If one option is given the probability value of 1 (occurring), the other will be given the probability value

Table 13.3 Types of data

Type of data	Example
Categorical	Eye color
Binomial	Sex
Ordinal	Likert scale
Interval	Number of students
Continuous	Weight

of 0 (not occurring). This makes it possible to perform logistic regression analysis for binary dependent outcome variables. *Ordinal data* has an order of ranks in its nature (like the Likert type questionnaire including very poor, poor, good, very good, and excellent). These can be ordered from 1 to 5. Ordinal data have an ordered nature of three or more levels. Nevertheless, the distances between these levels are not equal. The Anatomical Injury Scale (1–5), Injury Severity Score (1–75), and Glasgow Coma Scale (3–15) are examples of ordinal data. Ordinal data should be presented as median (range or interquartile range (IQR)). *Interval (discrete)* data are real whole numbers (like number of students in a college or number of road traffic collisions). They do not have decimal places. *Continuous data* are numerical or quantitative data that can take any value (like level of serum albumin, height, or stroke volume) and can take decimal places [6].

Two common mistakes in statistical analysis are considering ordinal data as continuous data, or changing the continuous data to ordinal data or categorical data in the research protocols. An example is changing the Glasgow Coma Scale to mild, moderate, and severe head injuries. Doing so will weaken the nature and strength of the analysis. It is advised to collect the actual ordinal or continuous data in the research protocols. It is always possible to change the ordinal or continuous data to categorical data during the analysis if needed but not the opposite.

13.4 Are the Data Normally Distributed?

It is essential to check for normality of continuous data before the analysis. This can be done by looking into the histograms [6]. Normal distribution should have a bell shape. This is important for deciding the form in which the data will be presented. If the data has a normal distribution, then it can be presented as mean (standard deviation/standard error of the mean) because the mean is the proper point-estimate. If the data are ordinal or do not have a normal distribution, then the median (interquartile range (IQR)) is the proper point-estimate as it lies in the middle of the data. Figure 13.1, which is in one of our recently published papers [7], highlights this point. It compares the New Injury Severity Score (NISS) of two independent groups. Since the data are ordinal, data were presented as box-and-whisker plot. The box represents the 25th to the 75th percentile IQR. Kindly note that the horizontal line within each box, which represents the median, is not in the middle, indicating that the data are not normal and skewed to the right.

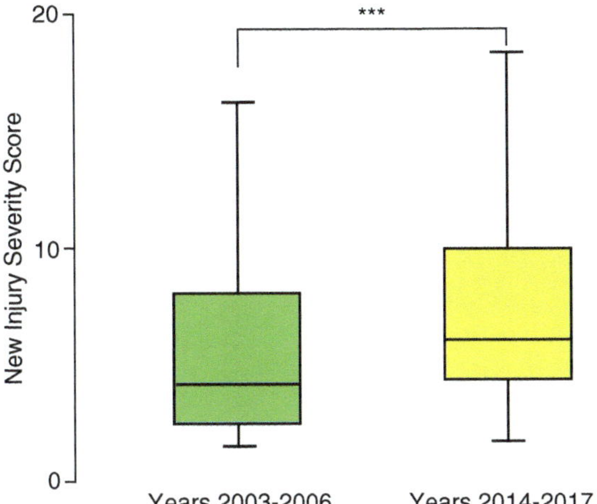

Fig. 13.1 Box-and-whisker plot of New Injury Severity Score (NISS) for hospitalized trauma patients during the period 2003–2006 (n = 2573) and 10 years later (n = 3519) during the period 2014–2017, Al-Ain Hospital, Al-Ain, United Arab Emirates. The box represents the 25th to the 75th percentile IQR. The horizontal line within each box represents the median. ***$p < 0.0001$, Mann–Whitney U test. (Reproduced from the study of Alao et al. [7]), which is distributed under the terms of the Creative Commons Attribution 4.0 International License)

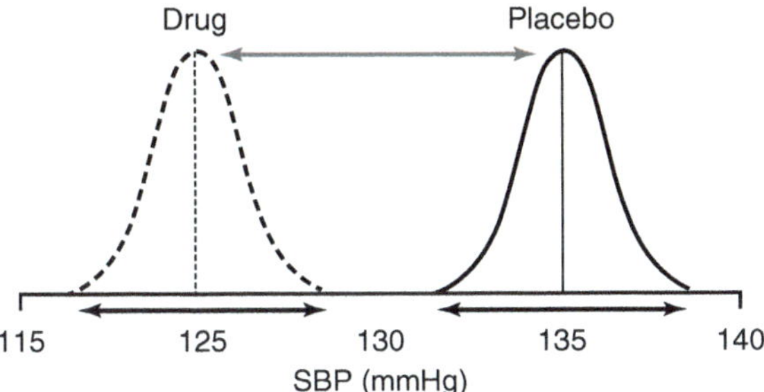

Fig. 13.2 A theoretical example testing a new anti-hypertensive drug. Hypertensive patients were randomized into two groups to receive the drug or a placebo. The data of both groups have a normal distribution and the variance of both groups (the black arrows) is equal. The difference between the means is 10 mmHg (gray arrow). The proper statistical test to use in this situation is the unpaired-t test (student's t test)

Comparing the continuous data of two groups using parametric methods requires two assumptions: (1) data should have a normal distribution, (2) data should have the same variability. Figure 13.2 is a theoretical example of testing a new anti-hypertensive drug. Hypertensive patients were randomized into two groups to receive the drug or a placebo, each having a sample of 200 subjects. Notice that the data of both groups have a normal distribution and the variance of both groups (the black arrows) is equal. The difference between the means is 10 mmHg (gray arrow). The proper statistical test to use in this situation is the unpaired-t test (student's t test).

The histogram can demonstrate whether the continuous data is skewed. If the data do not have a normal distribution, then there are two solutions: (1) change the data to normal distribution and then perform the analysis using a parametric method, define the mean of the new data, and then back transform it for reporting or (2) use non-parametric methods. As an example, Fig. 13.3 is retrieved from our recently published paper on the global data of motorcycle related death rates [8]. Kindly observe that the

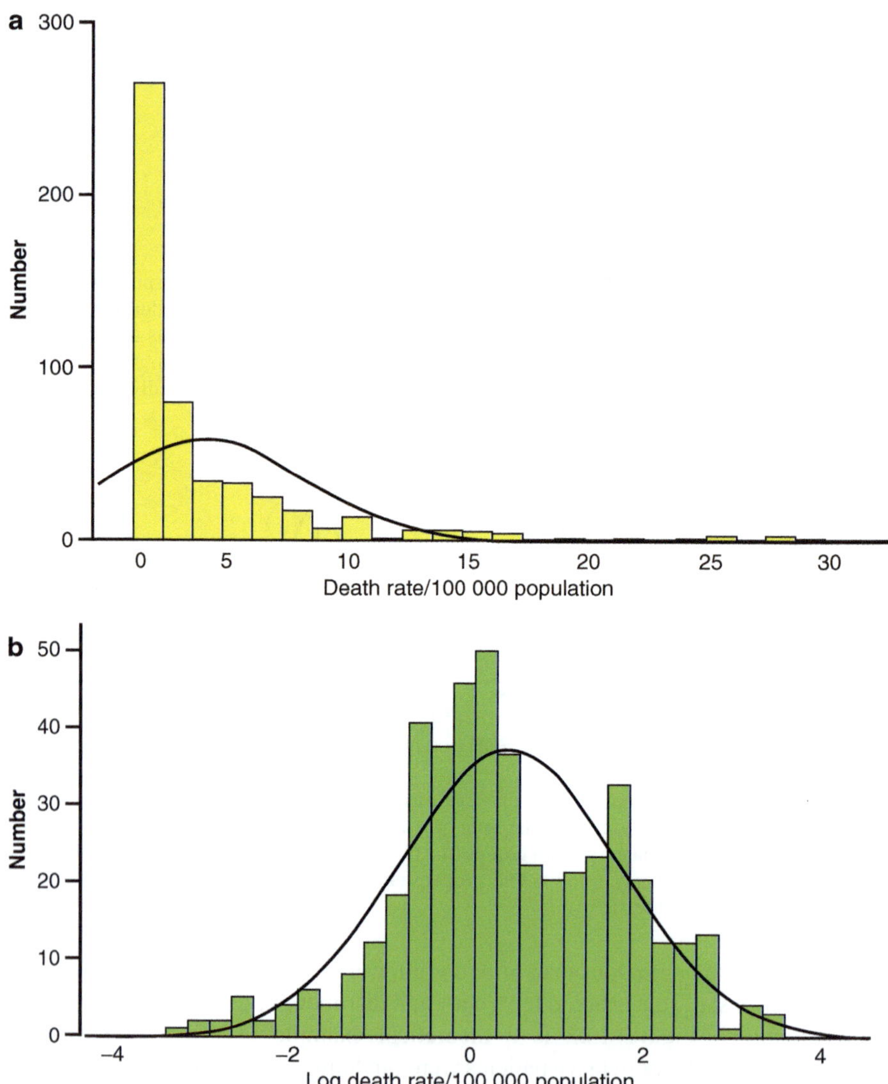

Fig. 13.3 Global data of motorcycle related death rates (**a**) and its log transformation (**b**) (crude data are from the study of Yasin et al. [8]), which is distributed under the terms of the Creative Commons Attribution 4.0 International License

data of death rates are skewed to the right (Fig. 13.3a) with a skewness value of 3.1 and having a wide peak (kurtosis) of 11.6. The normal values of both Skewness and kurtosis should be between −1 and 1 [6]. Log transformation of the data (Fig. 13.3b) has a normal distribution with skewness of −0.05 and kurtosis of 0.013. Accordingly, the log transformed data was used as the outcome variable in the mixed linear model. The outcome variable of mixed linear model should have a normal distribution.

13.5 How Many Groups Are Compared?

This question looks easy to answer but is sometimes tricky. We need to decide whether the data represent one group, two groups, or more than two groups in order to define the proper statistical method to be used. You should be careful differentiating between studied groups of patients and groups of data. You may measure a variable in one group of patients, give the same group a medication, and then measure the variable again after giving the medication. If the values of the variable are compared before and after the medication, these are two dependent groups of data although they were measured in the same group of patients.

13.6 What Is the Number of Subjects in Each Group?

Defining the size of subjects in each group is important to define the statistical methods of analysis. If the number of subjects is less than 20 in each group, it is advised to use non-parametric methods. Non-parametric methods compare the ranks, do not need a normal distribution, are useful in small samples, are more strict than parametric methods, and will not accept significance easily. One approach is to use non-parametric methods all the time, which I practice. There is a risk of missing statistical significance with this approach if parametric methods are not used in normal distributed data (type II statistical error). This may be important when trying to prove harm but not benefit. Kindly note that a significant *p* value in comparisons and correlations can be achieved when the sample size is very large. This may not translate to a clinically significant finding as the correlation may be weak or the effect size is small.

13.7 Are the Compared Data Related or Unrelated?

This question is very important and needs deep thinking to address. When comparing the weight of patients who died and those who survived following road traffic collisions, it is clear that these two groups are completely independent because each subject will be only in one group. In comparison, if we study the effect of bypass surgery on the weight of morbid obese patients, we will measure the weight before surgery and after surgery which enables us to measure weight change in each patient. Weight before surgery and after surgery are related (dependent) data. In the first example the two groups are independent and the weight of the two groups can

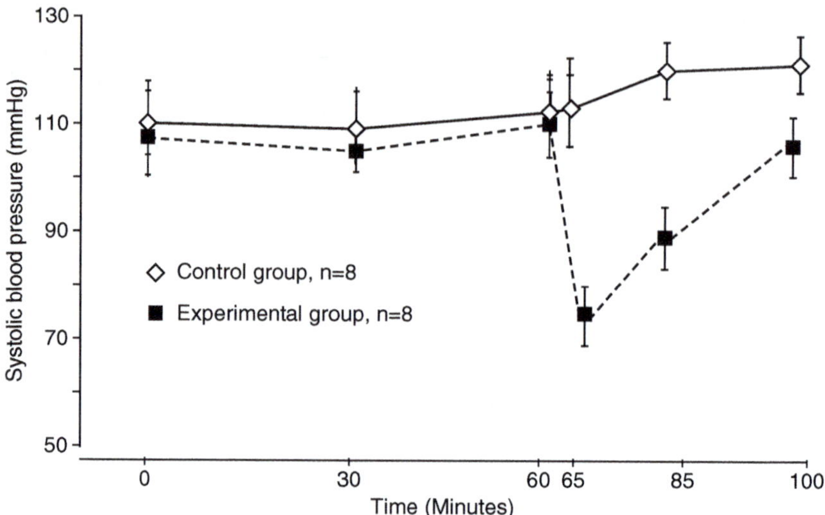

Fig. 13.4 A theoretical animal experiment comparing two groups of anesthetized rats, each consists of eight rats. One group is a control laparotomy group (white diamonds), while the other group is a bowel-ischemia reperfusion group (black square). The data presented are the mean systolic pressure (standard error of the mean) of each group over time. The proper method of statistical analysis in this situation is the repeated measurement analysis of variance

be compared using unpaired *t*-test if other assumptions of using this test were met. In the second example the two groups are dependent and the weight of the two groups can be compared using paired *t*-test. The paired *t*-test has the advantage of comparing each subject with itself which standardizes all variation within the subject and makes it easy to find the statistical significance. This analysis can be used in natural pairs like twins or selected matched pairs of patients.

Let us look into another common example. Figure 13.4 shows a theoretical animal experiment over time comparing two groups of anesthetized rats, each consists of eight rats. One group is a control laparotomy group (white diamonds), while the other group is a bowel-ischemia reperfusion group (black square). Systolic blood pressure (SBP) directly dropped following the small bowel reperfusion. Kindly note the relationship between the collected data of SBP. The data within each group are dependent as it is repeatedly measured in the same animal. In contrast, the data between the two groups are independent as each animal is located within a specific group. The proper method of statistical analysis in this situation is the repeated measurement analysis of variance. This analyzes three components: (1) difference within each group, (2) difference between groups, and (3) the interaction between the two groups to evaluate the direction of change. Each of these factors should have only a single reported p value [9–11].

13.8 Which Test to Use?

Table 13.4 shows the summary of the recommended statistical methods to be used for analyzing the continuous or ordinal data after answering the previous questions. We have now defined the type of data, number of the groups to be compared, number of the subjects within each group, whether the data have a normal distribution or not, and whether the data are related or not. Non-parametric statistical methods are the proper method when the number of the subjects of the groups are small, data do not have a normal distribution, or data are ordinal in nature. Non-parametric methods are advised in these conditions because they compare the ranks of the groups and a normal distribution is not needed [12, 13].

Let us assume that we are comparing the New Injury Severity Score (NISS) of trauma patients who were admitted during the last year in four different trauma centers in our state. Their numbers range between 750 and 1200 patients. The data are ordinal, the groups are independent, the number of the groups are more than 2. Then, the proper test to use is Kruskal–Wallis test. If the analysis was not significant, then we stop at this stage, and accept that the injury severity of the hospitalized trauma patients is the same between these four hospitals. If we find that there was statistical significance between the hospitals then we proceed with comparisons between each two hospitals using Mann–Whitney *U* test, just to explain the finding and not prove it, because the overall test will not be able to show that.

Beware that you should always use two tailed tests which indicate that the difference can go in any direction. This is the standard accepted way for comparison. Do not use a one tailed test. I have never used it in my three decades of intense research activities. One tailed test indicates that the difference between the groups can go only in one direction. This should be decided before the analysis is started, clearly mentioned and justified in the methods section, and clearly reported in the results section.

When comparing categorical data of two or more independent groups, then Pearson's Chi-square can be used. Nevertheless, if the sample size of the groups is small (less than 20), any of the cells is 0, or any of the expected cells is less than 5, then Fisher's Exact test should be used. Advanced Statistical packages (like SPSS, SPSS Inc, Chicago, IL, USA) will give a warning and advise which test is to be used. McNemar's test should be used when comparing matched (related) categorical data [14].

Table 13.4 Selection of statistical tests for comparison of continuous or ordinal data

	Parametric		Non-parametric	
	2 groups	>2 groups	2 groups	>2 groups
Independent	Unpaired *t*-test	ANOVA with multiple comparison Bonferroni correction	Mann–Whitney *U* test	Kruskal–Wallis test
Dependent	Paired *t*-test	Repeated measurement ANOVA	Wilcoxon Signed rank test	Friedman test

Do and Don't

- Understand the research question and the type of data thoroughly before starting the analysis.
- Define the number of groups to be compared, number of subjects in each group, and the relationship between the groups.
- Use parametric methods only for normally distributed data. Alternatively use non-parametric methods.
- Do not overuse statistics.
- Do not fish for a *p* value.
- Ask for help when needed.

Take Home Messages

- Basic statistics is easy to perform if well understood.
- There are two main types of statistical comparisons: parametric and non-parametric.
- The correct statistical method will be selected by following the roadmap explained in this chapter.

Conflict of Interest None declared by the author.

References

1. Sprent P. Statistics in medical research. Swiss Med Wkly. 2003;133(39–40):522–9.
2. Shaban S, Cevik AA, Canakci ME, Kuas C, El Zubeir M, Abu-Zidan F. Do senior medical students meet recommended emergency medicine curricula requirements? BMC Med Educ. 2018;18:8.
3. Ranganathan P, Pramesh CS, Buyse M. Common pitfalls in statistical analysis: the perils of multiple testing. Perspect Clin Res. 2016;7:106–7.
4. Yasin YJ, Alao DO, Grivna M, Abu-Zidan FM. Impact of the COVID-19 pandemic on road traffic collision injury patterns and severity in Al-Ain City, United Arab Emirates. World J Emerg Surg. 2021;16:57.
5. Hassard TH. Analysis of variance. In: Hassard TH, editor. Understanding biostatistics. 1st ed. St. Louis, MO: Mosby Year Book; 1991. p. 75–97.
6. Chan YH. Biostatistics 101: data presentation. Singapore Med J. 2003;44:280–5.
7. Alao DO, Cevik AA, Eid HO, Jummani Z, Abu-Zidan FM. Trauma system developments reduce mortality in hospitalized trauma patients in Al-Ain City, United Arab Emirates, despite increased severity of injury. World J Emerg Surg. 2020;15:49.
8. Yasin YJ, Grivna M, Abu-Zidan FM. Motorized 2-3 wheelers death rates over a decade: a global study. World J Emerg Surg. 2022;17:7.
9. Chan YH. Biostatistics 301. Repeated measurement analysis. Singapore Med J. 2004;45:354–68.
10. Munro BH. Repeated measures analysis of variance. In: Munro BH, editor. Statistical methods for health care research. 4th ed. New York: Lippincott; 2001. p. 201–21.
11. Ludbrook J. Repeated measurements and multiple comparisons in cardiovascular research. Cardiovasc Res. 1994;28:303–11.

12. Chan YH. Biostatistics 102: quantitative data—parametric & non-parametric tests. Singapore Med J. 2003;44:391–6.
13. Munro BH. Selected nonparametric techniques. In: Munro BH, editor. Statistical methods for health care research. 4th ed. New York: Lippincott; 2001. p. 97–121.
14. Chan YH. Biostatistics 103: qualitative data—tests of independence. Singapore Med J. 2003;44:498–503.

Further Reading

Guyatt G, Jaeschke R, Heddle N, Cook D, Shannon H, Walter S. Basic statistics for clinicians: 1. Hypothesis testing. CMAJ. 1995;152:27–32.

Hassard TH, editor. Understanding biostatistics. 1st ed. St. Louis, MO: Mosby Year Book; 1991.

Munro BH, editor. Statistical methods for health care research. 4th ed. New York: Lippincott; 2001.

Siegel S, Catellan NJ Jr. Nonparametric statistics for behavioral sciences. 2nd ed. Singapore: McGraw-Hill International Editions; 1988.

GPSR Compliance

The European Union's (EU) General Product Safety Regulation (GPSR) is a set of rules that requires consumer products to be safe and our obligations to ensure this.

If you have any concerns about our products, you can contact us on ProductSafety@springernature.com

In case Publisher is established outside the EU, the EU authorized representative is:

Springer Nature Customer Service Center GmbH
Europaplatz 3
69115 Heidelberg, Germany

Batch number: 10370712

Printed by Printforce, the Netherlands